帕金森病及其他运动障碍性疾病的经颅超声

张迎春 主 编

苏 州 大 学 出 版 社

图书在版编目(CIP)数据

帕金森病及其他运动障碍性疾病的经颅超声/张迎春主编.
—苏州:苏州大学出版社,2021.11(2023.3重印)
ISBN 978-7-5672-3729-2

Ⅰ.①帕… Ⅱ.①张… Ⅲ.①帕金森综合征—超声波疗法
②运动障碍—超声波疗法 Ⅳ.①R742.505②R749.505

中国版本图书馆 CIP 数据核字(2021)第 204956 号

帕金森病及其他运动障碍性疾病的经颅超声

张迎春　主编

责任编辑　李寿春

助理编辑　郭　佼

苏州大学出版社出版发行
(地址:苏州市十梓街 1 号　邮编:215006)
镇江文苑制版印刷有限责任公司印装
(地址:镇江市黄山南路 18 号润州花园 6-1　邮编:212000)

开本 787 mm×1 092 mm　1/32　印张 6.125　字数 100 千
2021 年 11 月第 1 版　2023 年 3 月第 2 次印刷
ISBN 978-7-5672-3729-2　定价:30.00 元

若有印装错误,本社负责调换
苏州大学出版社营销部　电话:0512-67481020
苏州大学出版社网址　http://www.sudapress.com
苏州大学出版社邮箱　sdcbs@suda.edu.cn

编 委 会

主　审：刘春风

主　编：张迎春

副主编：张　英　王才善　毛成洁

　　　　陈　静

编　委：（按姓氏拼音排序）

超声科

　　　　陈寒冰　陈晓芳　丁常伟

　　　　董智芬　傅心雨　郝丽君

　　　　李　晶　刘培青　刘松涛

　　　　毛　攀　盛爱妍　盛余敬

　　　　宋　馨　王才善　杨　敏

　　　　俞丽芳　张　英　张迎春

　　　　郑丽君　周　铭

磁共振室

范国华　蒋　震　王二磊

神经内科

陈　静　胡　华　罗蔚峰

毛成洁

睡眠中心

陈　锐

序言一

脑科学已成为国际研究重点与热点，世界主要国家纷纷投入巨资进行研究。《Science》杂志刊文也预测超声将在脑科学研究中发挥重要作用，但如何有效切入是我一直在思索的问题。

收到迎春主任对其新书《帕金森病及其他运动障碍性疾病的经颅超声》作序的邀请，很高兴，也很有感触！让我高兴的是，迎春主任的团队在帕金森病超声诊断方面做了大量的病例积累，她们的新书详细介绍了帕金森病的超声检查方法以及分期、分级方法，同时附上了相关国际诊断指南，是一本非常实用的书籍，我相信本书的出版一定会推动中国脑超声相关研究的进一步发展。让我感触的是，迎春主任团队所在的医院可能算不上国内的顶级医院，但他们能够写出这样一本好书，可见，只要敢想敢做，很多有理想有信念的超声人都可以在某些方面站在国内甚至国际的前沿。

我们生逢伟大的时代,面临世界百年未有之大变局,我相信,迎春主任的故事一定可以激发更多的超声人在各个超声亚专科领域取得令人瞩目的成绩,在捍卫人民生命健康的道路上,在实现第二个百年奋斗目标中,做出中国超声人的贡献!

郑元义

2021 年 10 月 11 日

(上海第六人民医院党委委员、副院长,中华医学会超声医学分会副主任委员、腹部组组长)

序言二

帕金森病是临床常见的神经退行性疾病，随着人口老龄化的加剧，其患病人数明显增加，但由于确切的发病机制尚不清楚，早期精准诊断和修饰治疗都很困难。

超声技术作为无创便捷的临床诊断技术，近年来在神经系统疾病的诊断中发挥着越来越大的作用。经颅超声多普勒技术广泛应用于脑血管疾病的诊疗过程中，而中脑黑质超声检查在帕金森病诊断中的应用也受到重视。我院超声中心张迎春主任自2009年起与神经内科团队合作，开展了超声技术在帕金森病诊断等方面应用的一系列研究工作，不仅建立了帕金森病相关的一套诊断操作流程和规范，还在肌张力障碍、原发性震颤、多系统萎缩、抑郁症、老年性痴呆等疾病患者中进行了系统观察，总结了这些疾病中颅脑超声的特异性表现，为这些疾病的诊断增加了一项无创检查手段。

虽然颅脑超声的发现还不能作为帕金森病的确诊指标，但为该病的诊断提供了很大的帮助，黑质强回声已经作为支持诊断的标准列入中国帕金森病诊断指南，随着临床证据的不断积累，其临床价值会不断提高。

为了推广经颅超声多普勒技术在帕金森病及其他运动障碍性疾病中的应用，张迎春主任组织编写了这本《帕金森病及其他运动障碍性疾病的经颅超声》，相信该书会为广大超声影像、神经内科和神经外科医师带来帮助。

刘春风

2021 年 10 月 19 日

（苏州大学神经研究所所长，苏州大学附属第二医院神经内科科主任、神经疾病研究中心主任）

前 言

2009年9月某一天,神经内科刘春风主任让罗蔚锋主任同我探讨:"据说超声可以检查帕金森病?"我一脸茫然:"不会吧?能查帕金森病的应该是经颅多普勒TCD吧?要不文献发我看看?"由此,我接触到了经颅超声检查的第一篇文献。读完那篇文献,我惭愧不已,作为一名超声科大夫,国外已经有了相关操作指南与规范,而我却一无所知!但同时,这一文献也使我内心一颗小火花跳跃起来——既然常规CT、MR对这疾病无特征性影像学表现,也许一把小小的超声探头,能够做点什么。

接下来的日子充实、辛苦和快乐。该领域的相关文献国内几乎没有,于是检索了几乎所有相关的国外文献,边临床边学习,解剖图对比着文献图,一个个核团摸索、确认,一份份病例沟通、随访。

一开始，临床答复常常是"这个黑质强回声，搞得我诊断都糊涂了！"渐渐地，临床反馈变为了"这个报告目前对我们诊断还是蛮有帮助的！"随着检查量逐年增加，我们的案例积累得越来越多，团队自信心慢慢建立了，人员也逐步壮大，临床水平日趋稳定。

帕金森病的临床异质性高，临床症状分为运动障碍、非运动障碍两大部分，具体又包括各种亚型，只能说这是一个太过狡猾的疾病！于是，团队针对该病不同的临床亚型，结合不同的检验指标和最新的诊断与鉴别诊断标准，利用各种超声新技术做了系统性研究。慢慢地，我明白了为什么不同文献报道的帕金森病患者黑质强回声比例不同，为什么欧美规范要这样建立，哪些核团容易混淆……

探索的过程离不开优秀文献的引导，Walter U、Daniela B、Berg D等教授的文章将我们一步步引入脑超的世界，并将我们探求之路上的疑团逐步解开。在多年的探索中，我们深深体会到文献学习和技术积累的重要性，也希望像帮助过我们的这些优秀学者那样，把知识的火炬传递下去，为医学的提升尽上绵薄之力。在这一初心的推动下，我们多次开办了经颅超声的学习班，推广新技术。课程上手把手带教时，学员们反复询问："有没有一本中文书籍可以供我们参考学习？"由此，产生了编书的想法。希望这本书，能够让初步开展经颅超声工作的同行们可以随时拿出来对照学习，可以通过这本书了解国外的规范指南，从而绕开那些我们曾经走过的弯路。

超声的主观性，必定是绕不过的话题。尤其对于颅内小小的核团，动辄以平方毫米为单位的面积描计，更需要我们掌握基本的解剖学知识和一定的操作技能。同时，由于欧亚人种的差异，临床上迫切需要建立起符合我国人群的经颅超声诊断规范与指南，我们任重道远。

《帕金森病及其他运动障碍性疾病的经颅超声》一书即将付梓，感谢编写组成员的辛勤付出，从五千多例资料中筛选出最清晰的图片用作插图，将多年的心得体会倾囊而出注于本书（第一章第一节由神经内科毛成洁及陈静负责编写；第一章第二节由影像磁共振室王二磊、范国华、蒋震负责编写；第二章及后面章节由超声科脑超团队成员、在读研究生及已毕业的脑超研究方向研究生合作完成）；感谢脑超团队多年的信任与团结合作，将最美的 12 年青春义无反顾地投入到这一领域；感谢主审刘春风教授的精心指导；感谢所有神经内科医生多年的默默支持；感谢中华超声医学会副主任委员、腹部及脑超组组长、上海六院郑元义教授的关心与大力支持！有了你们的帮助，经颅超声，道阻且长，行则将至，行而不辍，则未来可期。

苏州大学附属第二医院超声科　张迎春

2021 年 10 月 15 日

目录 Contents

第一章 帕金森病概述
第一节 帕金森病的临床诊断……………… 1

第二节 帕金森病磁共振成像技术研究进展
………………………………… 17

第二章 经颅超声概论 …………………… 30

第三章 帕金森病经颅超声相关研究 ………… 43
第一节 帕金森病与经颅超声 …………… 43

第二节 帕金森病运动症状与经颅超声
………………………………… 51

第三节 帕金森病非运动症状与经颅超声
………………………………… 55

第四章 其他运动障碍性疾病与经颅超声 …… 76
第一节 原发性震颤 …………… 76
第二节 多系统萎缩 …………… 83
第三节 肌张力障碍 …………… 87

第五章 经颅超声的临床实践 ………… 95

附 录 …………………………… 100
附录一 帕金森病的经颅超声检查操作规范流程 ………… 100
附录二 苏州大学附属第二医院 TCS 检查报告模板 ………… 113
附录三 欧美 TCS 检查规范（2014 版） ………… 115
附录四 不同临床疾病经颅超声检查表现 ………… 162
附录五 中国帕金森病的诊断标准（2016 版） ………… 163
附录六 缩略词表 ………… 177

第一章 帕金森病概述

第一节 帕金森病的临床诊断

帕金森病（Parkinson's disease，PD）是最常见的神经系统退行性疾病之一，年平均发病率为14/10万人，65岁以上人群的年发病率为160/10万人。目前全球有600多万名帕金森病患者，其主要的临床表现为静止性震颤、运动迟缓、肌强直和姿势步态的异常等。此外，还包括一些非运动症状，如快速眼动睡眠期行为障碍、自主神经功能障碍、焦虑和抑郁等。

帕金森病有多种亚型，不同亚型预后各有差异，主要分为三种亚型。最常见的为轻度运动为主型，约占帕金森病的49%~53%，这一类型起病早，运动症状较轻，对多巴胺能药物反应良好且疾病进展缓慢。其次为中间型，约占帕金森病的

35%~39%，起病年龄中等，运动症状介于其余两型之间，对多巴胺能药物反应尚可且疾病进展中等。最少见的为弥漫恶化型，占帕金森病的9%~16%，这一类型早期有明显的运动和非运动症状，对药物反应不良且疾病进展更快[1]。

帕金森病的治疗主要以对症治疗为主，重点是改善运动症状（如静止性震颤、肌强直、运动迟缓等）和非运动症状（如便秘、认知障碍、情绪不稳定、睡眠障碍等），目前还没有阻止病情发展的特效药物。多巴胺能药物治疗通常可帮助改善最初的运动症状，而非运动性症状需要非多巴胺能途径的治疗方法（如选择性5-羟色胺再摄取抑制剂用于精神症状的治疗，胆碱酯酶抑制剂用于认知障碍的治疗等）。康复治疗和运动治疗是药物治疗的补充。中晚期帕金森病患者会出现一些运动并发症，如症状波动、异动症及肌张力障碍等。存在并发症的帕金森病患者可接受一些更为先进的治疗方法，如左旋多巴-卡比多巴肠溶悬液治疗或脑深部电刺激术的治疗等。

帕金森病虽然特征明显，但仍需要由神经科医师依据临床表现，结合辅助检查，并进行有效的鉴别诊断后进行合理诊断，其中准确的病史采集、仔细的体格检查以及合理的辅助检查十分重要。

一、帕金森病的诊断方法

1. 病史

病史在帕金森病的诊断中非常重要。帕金森病多见于中老年人群，常隐袭起病，其运动症状主要有静止性震颤、运动迟缓、肌强直和姿势平衡障碍。同时，也会有一些前驱期症状或者非运动症状，包括嗅觉障碍、睡眠障碍、便秘、多汗、流涎、排尿困难、性功能减退、幻觉、疼痛、焦虑抑郁等。另外，帕金森病患者对于药物的反应也有助于疾病的诊断。

2. 体格检查

神经系统体格检查对帕金森病的诊断及鉴别诊断非常重要。如发现静止性震颤、铅管样或齿轮样肌张力增高，更多考虑诊断帕金森病；如角膜发现K-F环则通常提示肝豆状核变性。精神和智能检查可发现精神疾病及其他的神经变性疾病，如亨廷顿舞蹈病和肝豆状核变性等常伴有精神和智能损害。醉酒步态、直立性低血压，须考虑脊髓小脑性共济失调、多系统萎缩等。

3. 辅助检查

合理的辅助检查有助于将帕金森病与其他运动障碍性疾病进行有效鉴别。临床中比较常见的辅助检查有：血清铜、尿铜和血清铜蓝蛋白含量测定，可帮助诊断肝豆状核变性；头颅 MRI 可发现小脑萎缩、中脑萎缩及基底节异常信号等；头颅 CT 可发现肝豆状核变性患者的双侧豆状核区低密度灶；SPECT 或 PET 可显示帕金森病患者纹状体多巴胺转运体功能降低、多巴胺合成减少和 D_2 型多巴胺受体（D_2R）活性改变；经颅超声可发现黑质异常强回声等。此外，对于某些具有家族史或特殊表型的患者，基因检测也具有一定的诊断价值。

4. 帕金森病诊断流程图

2016 年国际帕金森病及运动障碍学会以及我国帕金森病及运动障碍学组和专委会制定了《中国帕金森病的诊断标准（2016 版）》，里面包含了帕金森病的诊断标准、支持标准、排除标准、警示征象[2-4]。上述标准是对帕金森病病史采集、体格检查以及辅助检查的具体细化及概括总结，以进一步帮助医师对帕金森病进行准确诊断，其诊断流程图如下（图1-1）：

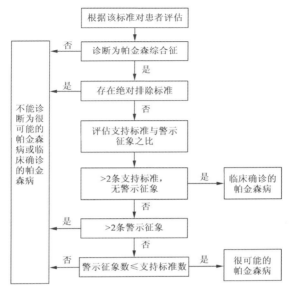

图1-1 帕金森病诊断流程图

注：本图来自《中华神经科杂志》，2016，49（4）：268-271.

二、帕金森病的相关诊断标准

1. 帕金森病的诊断标准（必备条件）

a. 运动迟缓：即运动缓慢和在持续运动中运动幅度或速度的下降；

b. 至少存在静止性震颤或肌强直中的一项。

上述2条是诊断帕金森病的必备条件。

2. 帕金森病的支持标准（支持条件）

a. 多巴胺能药物有明确疗效；

b. 出现左旋多巴引起的异动症；

c. 可观察到患者单个肢体的静止性震颤；

d. 辅助检查提示：嗅觉减退或消失；或头颅超声显示黑质异常高回声（$\geqslant 20 \text{ mm}^2$）；或心脏间碘苄胍（MIBG）闪烁显像法显示心脏去交感神经支配。

上述标准是诊断帕金森病的支持条件，符合的条目越多，越支持帕金森病的诊断。

3. 帕金森病的排除标准（不应存在下列情况）

a. 存在明确小脑受损的体征；

b. 出现向下的垂直性核上性凝视麻痹，或眼睛向下扫视时速度减慢；

c. 起病 5 年内，高度怀疑为行为变异型额颞叶痴呆或原发性进行性失语；

d. 起病 3 年后，帕金森症状仍局限在下肢；

e. 服过多巴胺受体阻滞剂或多巴胺耗竭类药物，且药物剂量和服用时间与药物性帕金森综合征发病相符；

f. 中等严重程度的病情时，对大剂量左旋多巴治疗反应不明显；

g. 明确的皮层复合感觉缺失，或存在肢体观念运动性失用，或进行性失语；

h. 分子神经影像学检查突触前多巴胺系统功能正常；

i. 有其他的可以解释患者目前帕金森症状的其他疾病；或者本领域专家判断其可能为其他综合征，而非帕金森病。

上述标准是医生鉴别帕金森病与其他疾病的重要指标，医生诊断帕金森病时，需要依据上述情况进行排除。

4. 帕金森病的警示征象（支持判断其他疾病）

a. 发病 5 年内迅速出现严重的步态障碍，以至于需要经常使用轮椅；

b. 除去药物调整的因素，病情在 5 年内或 5 年以上稳定不进展；

c. 发病 5 年内出现严重的构音障碍、吞咽障碍；

d. 发病 5 年内出现吸气性呼吸功能障碍；

e. 发病 5 年内出现严重的自主神经功能障碍，包括：体位性低血压，严重的尿潴留或尿失禁；

f. 发病 3 年内出现明显的平衡功能障碍，导致反复跌倒（>1 次/年）；

g. 发病10年内出现不成比例的颈部前倾或手足挛缩；

h. 发病5年内不出现常见的非运动症状；

i. 出现其他原因不好解释的锥体束征；

g. 发病后帕金森症状始终为双侧对称。

上述标准是鉴别帕金森病与其他疾病的重要指标，符合的条目越多，越支持诊断为其他疾病。

三、帕金森病的鉴别诊断

1. 进行性核上性麻痹（progressive supranuclear palsy，PSP）

进行性核上性麻痹是一种常见的运动不能-肌强直综合征，每100位诊断为帕金森病的患者中，可能有5位是进行性核上性麻痹。除了帕金森病的主要症状如肌强直、运动缓慢和姿势不稳外，进行性核上性麻痹患者还存在眼睛活动障碍，主要是垂直方向眼球活动受限，还常有明显平衡障碍，因此他们经常跌倒。与帕金森病患者不同，进行性核上性麻痹患者的跌倒通常是一个早期而非晚期症状，而且是身体向后跌倒。进行性核上性麻痹通常以中轴症状为主，无震颤发生，对药物敏感性差。同时，患者有不能控制的鼓掌征，表现为连续鼓掌次数超过要求次数，停不住。头部 MRI 可有中脑萎缩。疾病的进展较帕金森病更快。

2. 多系统萎缩（multiple system atrophy，MSA）

多系统萎缩与帕金森病相似，通常无震颤发生，对药物敏感性差或无效，病情进展比帕金森病快。疾病早期就有明显的自主神经系统损害的症状，如直立低血压、尿失禁、性功能障碍等。有些患者查体可有锥体束征，可有吸气性喘鸣、早期颈项前屈等。多系统萎缩分两个亚型。① MSA-P 亚型与帕金森病症状非常相似，但对帕金森病药物不敏感、肌强直运动减少多对称。MSA-P 亚型患者静止性震颤少见，多见不规则、高频姿势性震颤等。② MSA-C 亚型主要表现为行走和平衡的困难、共济失调很明显、宽基步态等。多系统萎缩患者头部 MRI 检查可见脑桥部"十字征"、小脑萎缩等。

3. 皮质基底节变性（corticobasal degeneration，CBD）

皮质基底节变性与进行性核上性麻痹相似，但不同的是进行性核上性麻痹同时开始于两侧，皮质基底节变性首先开始于一侧，且皮质基底节变性比进行性核上性麻痹更易出现肌强直。进行性核上性麻痹患者的眼球运动总是受到影响，而皮质基底节变性患者的眼球运动可能不受影响，在皮质基底节变性和进行性核上性麻痹中跌倒都很常见。每100位帕金森病患者中可能有1位是皮质基底节变性，在尸检时皮质基底节变性与进行性核上性麻痹相似但不同于帕金森病和多系统萎缩。皮质基底节变性患者多有大脑皮质受损的表现（如复合感觉障碍、失用症等），查体可有锥体束征。头部MRI可见非对称性顶叶萎缩等。

4. 特发性震颤（essential tremor，ET）

特发性震颤又叫原发性震颤，是很常见的运动障碍疾病。原发性震颤的发病率比帕金森病的发病率高10~20倍，往往具有家族史。原发性震颤主要影响手，对头和足的影响相对少一些，震颤在注意力集中、精神紧张、疲劳、饥饿时加重，多数病例在饮酒后暂时消失，次日加重。与帕金森病不同，原发性震颤同时开始于两侧手，而且原发性震颤的震颤出现于手部运动的时候，这与帕金森病不同。一般情况下，帕金森病药物不会改善原发性震颤症状，原发性震颤对一些药物如扑痫酮（抗癫痫药）、普萘洛尔（用于治疗高血压的药）和苯二氮卓类药物（治疗焦虑的药）敏感，而这与帕金森病不同。

5. 其他

另外，还有路易体痴呆、脊髓小脑性共济失调、药物性帕金森综合征、肝豆状核变性、肌张力障碍、基底节区脑梗死、外伤等疾病均可表现出帕金森病样症状，在临床诊治过程中需要进行鉴别。

四、帕金森病的辅助检查

虽然有很多的影像技术都对帕金森病的诊断有一定帮助，但到目前为止还没有特定的检测方法来进行确诊[5]。询问包括症状及各种症状彼此之间的关系及其演变的病史，并进行神经科检查，是目前做出诊断的重要方法。

1. 头部 MRI 检查

MRI 也就是磁共振成像，它利用磁共振现象从人体中获得电磁信号，并重建出人体信息。头部 MRI 并不能诊断帕金森病，但可以帮助排除一些疾病，如多发性脑梗死、脑积水、肝豆状核变性、脊髓小脑性共济失调、多系统萎缩等，而这些疾病可与帕金森病症状相似。头部 MRI 检查是医生进行鉴别诊断的必要参考。

2. 头部 PET 检查

PET 即正电子发射型计算机断层显像，是核医学领域比较先进的临床检查影像技术。其是将某种物质，一般是生命代谢中必需的物质，如葡萄糖、蛋白质、核酸、脂肪酸等，标记上短寿命的放射性核素（如18F、11C等），注入人体后，通过该物质在代谢中的聚集情况，来反映生命代谢活动的情况，从而达到诊断的目的。帕金森病的PET检查一般选用3种。① DAT显像：DAT是多巴胺能神经元突触前膜的一种膜蛋白，它可以在多巴胺能神经元发放神经冲动后把突触间隙的多巴胺转运回突触前膜再利用或进一步分解，因此可以影响多巴胺的浓度。它的数量与多巴胺能神经元数量，能够直接反映突触前膜多巴胺能神经元的变化，比突触后膜的多巴胺受体变化更早、更直接、更敏感。由于多巴胺能神经元的减少和DAT数量减少正相关，两者相关性较好，即使替代治疗使患者症状改善，DAT也进行性、不可逆地下降，这与帕金森病病情不可逆进展的特点相符合。② 18F-dopa显像：反映的是黑质纹状体突触前多巴脱羧酶的活性，该酶的活性与多巴胺能神经元数目密切相关。帕金森病患者多巴胺合成减少，因此18F-dopa显像可反映基底多巴胺代谢情况。③ 18F-FDG（18F-脱氧葡萄糖）显像：脑以葡萄糖作为最主要能源，因此葡萄糖代谢可反映脑内神经元的活性，帕金森病患者 18F-FDG 显像的原理是患者多巴胺能神经元变性缺失、神经元数量减少导致能量需求降低，对葡萄糖摄取减少，因此葡萄糖代谢降低。头部 PET 检查是相对较特异的诊断帕金森病的辅助检查。

3. 经颅超声检查

经颅超声（transcranial sonography，TCS）作为一种新型的神经系统影像学检查方法，可以追溯到二十世纪七八十年代。经颅超声检查与常规的影像检查技术 CT、MRI 相比，操作简便，耗时短，被检者无须特殊准备。经颅超声能够通过颞窗获取中脑、丘脑等大脑深部组织结构的高分辨率图像，可提供脑黑质功能状态不可多得的信息。自 1995 年 Becker 等人首次报道应用经颅超声探及帕金森病患者中脑黑质存在特异性强回声以来，该技术引起国内外学者的广泛关注。目前，经颅超声检查技术已经成为欧美国家检查运动障碍性疾病的首选方式之一。大量研究表明 50%~90% 的帕金森病患者经颅超声检查会出现黑质强回声，而在帕金森综合征、原发性震颤等患者中却很少发现（图 1-2）。

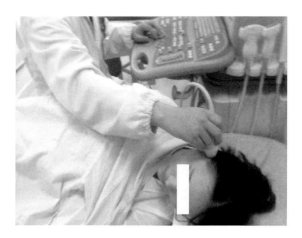

(a)

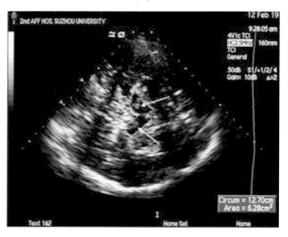

(b)

图 1-2 经颅超声检查（a）及黑质强回声图像（b）

经颅超声检查是医生诊断帕金森病重要的辅助检查手段。

4. 基因检测

自从1997年对SNCA突变的认识以来，对帕金森病基因突变的认识更加深入，目前已经证实的PD致病基因有20余个，包括常染色体显性遗传致病基因（LRRK2、SNCA等）、常染色体隐性遗传致病基因（PARK2、PINK1、DJ-1等）及X连锁致病基因等。还有许多风险基因或多态性位点被报道与PD相关，这进一步提示遗传因素在PD研究中的重要性。不同的基因其表型不同，例如Parkin突变的患者首发症状多为震颤（65%）和运动迟缓（63%），发病年龄早（大多数病人发病<40岁），病情进展缓慢，病程长，左旋多巴所致的剂末效应、开关现象、异动症等药物副反应较常见。Parkin基因突变的患者更易有冲动控制障碍。LRRK2基因突变的患者通常发病年龄较晚，病程长，药物剂量相对来说更大，但在嗅觉、焦虑抑郁、认知功能等非运动症状方面与Parkin基因突变的患者并没有明显的差距。GBA基因突变的患者认知功能障碍、痴呆和幻觉的频率要明显高于非携带者。SNCA基因突变的PD患者震颤的发生率

较低，但发病年龄更早且病程进展更快，同时会伴有痴呆、低血压、自主神经功能障碍、嗅觉减退以及快速眼动睡眠期行为障碍，并且嗅觉减退以及快速眼动睡眠期行为障碍通常是先于运动症状出现的。

5. 其他检查

目前，暂没有实验室检查能直接确诊帕金森病。临床检验中，有些检查可以帮助进行鉴别诊断。实验室指标中血清铜、尿铜和血清铜蓝蛋白含量测定可帮助诊断肝豆状核变性；血液异常红细胞（红细胞表面有棘状突起，称为棘红细胞）可帮助诊断棘红细胞增多症；脑脊液检查可以明确颅内感染情况，帮助诊断脑炎。

有些研究提示帕金森病患者血尿酸水平可有降低；脑脊液中可检出多巴胺水平降低，其代谢产物高香草酸浓度降低；有些帕金森病患者脑脊液中α-Syn、tau蛋白水平有改变。目前上述指标多处于研究阶段，尚未在临床检验中开展具体应用。

参考文献

[1] ARMSTRONG M J, OKUN M S. Diagnosis and

treatment of Parkinson disease: A review[J]. JAMA, 2020, 323 (6): 548-560.

[2] POSTUMA R B, BERG D, STERM M, et al. MDS clinical diagnostic criteria for Parkinson's disease[J]. Movement Disorders, 2015, 30(12): 1591-1601.

[3] 中华医学会神经病学分会帕金森病及运动障碍学组, 中国医师协会神经内科医师分会帕金森病及运动障碍专业委员会. 中国帕金森病的诊断标准（2016版）[J]. 中华神经科杂志, 2016, 49（4）: 268-271.

[4] SEPPI K, CHAUDHURI K R, COEIHOM, et al. Update on treatments for nonmotor symptoms of Parkinson's disease-an evidence-based medicine review[J]. Mov Disord, 2019, 34(2): 180-198.

[5] 崔海伦, 张一帆, 管晓军, 等. 帕金森病及相关运动障碍的神经影像学诊断专家共识[J]. 内科理论与实践, 2018, 13（5）: 320-324.

第二节 帕金森病磁共振成像技术研究进展

近些年来，磁共振成像（magnetic resonance imaging, MRI）检查由于其空间分辨率高、无创性、无辐射、检查方法多样化等优点而应用广泛，其在帕金森病的研究中有诸多应用。随着高场（3.0 T或以上）磁共振的普及，图像信噪比和对比度得到了很大程度的提高。一些新的成像序列、相关后处理技术及指标的开发为探究帕金森病的神经病理机制提供了新思路。

一、结构磁共振成像技术在帕金森病中的应用

近年来，结构磁共振成像技术凭借其高对比度（灰质、白质及脑脊液的信号对比度高）和高分辨率（1 mm×1 mm×1 mm）的特点，为探究帕金森病患者大脑病理结构变化提供了客观的评估手段。目前，针对结构磁共振成像的后处理分析方法及指标主要包括：基于体素的形态学分析方法（voxel-based morphometry，VBM）、皮层厚度（cortical thickness，CT）和一系列皮层形态学指标，如局部分形维数（local fractal dimension，LFD）、局部回指数（local gyrification index，LGI）及沟深（sulcal depth，SD）等。

基于体素的形态学分析方法和皮层厚度测量是目前使用最广泛的两种方法。目前许多相关研究均

发现帕金森病患者存在广泛的灰质体积萎缩及皮层厚度变薄[1-4]，这些脑区涉及额叶、颞叶、顶叶、枕叶、岛叶、深部核团及小脑等。但只能反映灰质的体积变化，无法显示大脑表面皮层形态的改变。

局部分形维数是一个新的定量评估皮层表面复杂程度改变的指标。大脑皮层的局部分形维数可以看作是皮层折叠频率、脑沟深度及脑回旋转的集合。目前研究发现帕金森病患者存在广泛的脑区局部分形维数降低，包括左侧的中央前回、中央后回、额上回、额中回后部、双侧的顶上回及右侧的颞上回等，且左侧中央后回的局部分形维数值与帕金森病病程呈显著负相关。左侧中央后回属于感觉运动区，这可能解释了这些患者进展性的平衡能力减退及加重的步态困难[5]。

局部回指数是一个在顶点水平定量评估皮层折叠程度的指标，反映一定区域内包埋在脑沟内的皮层与大脑表面皮层的比值。目前研究发现帕金森病晚期（病程>5年）的患者也存在部分脑区局部回指数降低，包括双侧的顶下小叶、中央前回、中央后回、额上回及缘上回，并且随访研究发现上述脑区的局部回指数值随着帕金森病病程的延长而逐渐降低[6]。

沟深是基于欧氏距离的脑沟软脑膜面（内表面）到外表面的直线距离。研究发现帕金森病患者较正常对照组存在额颞顶枕及岛叶等广泛脑区的沟深减低，并且左侧额下回三角部的沟深值降低可以预测帕金森病患者认知损害程度[7]。

根据帕金森病的 Braak 病理分级：疾病早期路易体病理改变局限于脑干、延髓、嗅球及黑质等部位，随着病情进展逐渐累及大脑皮层，其中，最先累及颞叶和旧皮质区（4级），然后是额叶和高级感觉联合皮层（5级），最后累及运动前区和中央前后回等感觉运动区（6级）[8]。路易体病理改变造成神经元的凋亡，可以引起脑结构的萎缩改变。因此通过高分辨结构像磁共振成像，我们可以从灰质体积、皮层厚度及皮层形态学等多个角度对帕金森病患者的宏观脑结构改变进行客观的评估，这为探究帕金森病严重程度及监测疾病进展提供了重要手段。

二、磁共振铁成像技术在帕金森病中的应用

帕金森病的病理特征是黑质致密部多巴胺能神经元的缺失和 α-突触核蛋白的异常聚集形成的路

易体病理。黑质区域内铁的过度沉积可以导致氧化应激损伤和促进α-突触核蛋白聚集,从而加重多巴胺能神经元的凋亡,因此对帕金森病患者铁的定量评估具有早期诊断和监测疾病进展的意义。近年来,磁共振铁成像技术不断发展,磁敏感加权成像(susceptibility weighted imaging,SWI)正是基于铁沉积导致的组织磁化率差异的一种磁共振铁成像技术,但是容易受到感兴趣区几何形状和方向的影响,且结果仅为一种半定量测定。而定量磁敏感成像(quantitative susceptibility mapping,QSM)是近年来基于磁敏感加权成像技术发展而来的一项新的磁共振铁成像技术。该技术通过将相位信息转化成局部性磁化率来定量铁含量,具有较高的敏感度和分辨度,因此得到了广泛的认可和应用。采用这两种技术,研究者发现了帕金森病患者黑质小体-1"燕尾征"的消失,这对鉴别帕金森病患者和正常人具有较高的敏感性[9]。研究者利用定量磁敏感成像技术发现帕金森病患者黑质、红核、丘脑底核和苍白球的定量磁敏感值较正常对照者明显增高,且黑质、红核和苍白球的定量磁敏感值与帕金森病H-Y分期呈显著正相关[10]。另外,帕金森病伴轻度认知障碍的患者较不伴轻度认知障碍的患者在楔叶、楔前叶、尾状核头、梭状回、眶额皮层、内嗅皮层、海马旁回及杏仁核的定量磁敏感值显著增高，且上述部分脑区与蒙特利尔认知评估量表（Monotreal cognitive assessment，MoCA）评分呈显著负相关，这些结果均表明认知损害会加重帕金森病患者的脑铁沉积，定量铁沉积测定能够预测认知损害程度[11]，具有较高的可靠性和敏感性。

三、磁共振扩散成像技术在帕金森病中的应用

磁共振扩散成像技术被广泛用于探测生物组织微观结构特性及大脑结构连通性、评价神经组织的微观结构。扩散张量成像（diffusion tensor imaging，DTI）是使用最广泛的扩散成像技术，能够无创性显示脑白质纤维的微观结构、形态及密度等信息。其扩散参数部分如各向异性、平均扩散率、轴向扩散率和径向扩散率等可以对脑白质纤维进行量化，反映其内在的细微结构变化。以往大量扩散张量成像研究发现了帕金森病患者存在广泛脑区的白质损害，包括胼胝体、小脑、上纵束和下纵束等[12]。但仅仅只能描述脑白质结构，不能全面地解释交叉和分叉白质纤维结构。近年来，优化的扩散成像技

术，如扩散峰度成像技术和神经突方向离散度与密度成像技术提供了新的度量指标，如轴向峰度、径向峰度、平均峰度、神经突起内容积比、方向离散度和各向同性间隔的体积分数等，这有利于提高诊断的敏感性及准确率[13]。

四、静息态功能磁共振成像技术在帕金森病中的应用

通过对与神经活动有关的大脑血氧水平依赖性的评测，静息态功能磁共振成像（resting-state functional magnetic resonance imaging，RS-fMRI）技术可以无创、间接地探测全脑神经活动，该技术只须受试者保持安静不动，无须复杂的任务态配合，因此得到了广泛应用。目前静息态功能磁共振的分析方法有局部一致性、低频振幅、独立成分分析、静态及动态功能连接等。通过应用这些方法，大量的研究发现帕金森病涉及多个脑网络内及之间的功能连接异常，如默认网络内功能连接的减低在帕金森病认知损害中发挥了重要作用[14]、以岛叶为中心的凸显网络与执行控制网络的连接中断可能是帕金森病伴抑郁的潜在发生机制[15]。尽管静息态功能磁共振在帕金森病的研究中得到了广泛应用，但是由于不同研究采用的样本量大小、被试特征、扫描设备及分析方法的不同，造成结果的可重复性比较差，所以仍需要标准化的技术和方法来提升其临床应用价值。

五、图论分析方法在帕金森病中的应用

近年来，利用图论分析方法对大脑进行大尺度网络分析在神经影像领域应用越来越广泛。人类的大脑可看作是一个复杂网络，由多个相互连接的脑区组成。每个脑区为一个网络节点，脑区之间的连接被定义为边，从而可以采用一系列指标对大脑的拓扑属性改变进行定量探究。图论分析方法与结构磁共振成像技术、扩散成像技术和静息态功能磁共振成像技术的结合研究，已表明帕金森病患者存在大尺度的脑网络连接异常。与正常对照者相比，帕金森病患者的脑网络存在次优的拓扑组织，导致大脑区域间信息整合能力降低[16-18]。图论的分析方法为我们探究帕金森病患者的神经病理改变机制提供了大尺度网络水平的新视角。

六、机器学习在帕金森病中的应用

近年来，机器学习（machine learning，ML）

方法在帕金森病中的应用愈加广泛。目前基于机器学习的神经影像分析流程主要包含特征提取、特征选择、训练分类、泛化能力测试等,其中特征选择及分类方法的多样性为机器学习模型的优化提供了更多的可能性[19-21]。机器学习与磁共振成像技术(如结构磁共振成像技术、扩散成像技术和静息态功能磁共振成像技术等)的紧密结合,为疾病的准确分类、预测及影像标志物识别开辟了有效途径。例如,对结构磁共振成像的灰白质体积、皮层厚度和面积等及静息态功能磁共振成像的局部一致性、低频振幅、功能连接和网络属性等特征指标的单独或融合应用,有助于对帕金森病患者与健康人群对照,或进行类似疾病的正确识别和分类,发现分类效能最高的异常特征脑区,加深对疾病的了解。在未来的研究中,我们应更加重视多模态磁共振成像技术在帕金森病前驱期的应用,它可以提供关于大脑结构及功能变化的多方面信息,提高模型的分类效能,有望成为帕金森病自动诊断、综合评价及机制研究的有力工具[22,23]。

七、小结

综上所述,磁共振多样化的成像技术及分析方法的应用为探究帕金森病神经病理机制提供了较为理想的工具,将有助于帕金森病的早期诊断、病情随访及疗效评估。

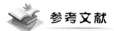
参考文献

[1] ZHENG D, CHEN C, SONG W C, et al. Regional gray matter reductions associated with mild cognitive impairment in Parkinson's disease: A meta-analysis of voxel-based morphometry studies[J]. Behav Brain Res, 2019, 371: 111973.

[2] BLAIR J C, BARRETT M J, PATRIE J, et al. Brain MRI reveals ascending atrophy in Parkinson's disease across severity[J]. Frontiers in Neurology, 2019, 10: 1329-1344.

[3] GAO Y Y, KUN N, MEI M J, et al. Changes in cortical thickness in patients with early Parkinson's disease at different Hoehn and Yahr stages[J]. Front Hum Neurosci, 2018, 12: 469.

[4] URIBE C, SEGURA B, BAGGIO H C, et al. Cortical atrophy patterns in early Parkinson's disease patients using hierarchical cluster analysis[J]. Parkinsonism Relat Disord, 2018, 50: 3-9.

[5] LI D, WANG E L, JIA Y J, et al. Cortical complexity and gyrification patterns in Parkinson's disease[J]. Neuroreport,

2020, 31(7): 565-570.

[6] NICHOLAS W, WANG M, ZHANG L J, et al. Stage-dependent loss of cortical gyrificationas Parkinson disease "unfolds"[J]. Neurology, 2016, 86(12): 1143-1151.

[7] WANG E, JIA Y J, YA Y, et al. Patterns of sulcal depth and cortical thickness in Parkinson's disease[J]. Brain Imaging and Behavior, 2021, 5月21日网上称发未见于纸刊.

[8] BRAAK H, TREDICI K D, RUB U, et al. Staging of brain pathology related to sporadic Parkinson's disease[J]. Neurobiology of Aging, 2003, 24(2): 197-211.

[9] CHENG Z H, HE N Y, HUANG P, et al. Imaging the nigrosome 1 in the substantia nigra using susceptibility weighted imaging and quantitative susceptibility mapping: an application to Parkinson's disease[J]. Neuroimage Clin, 2020, 25: 102-103.

[10] SHAHMAEI V, FAEGHI F, MOHAMMDBEIGI A, et al. Evaluation of iron deposition in brain basal ganglia of patients with Parkinson's disease using quantitative susceptibility mapping[J]. Eur J Radiol Open, 2019, 6: 169-174.

[11] UCHIDA Y, KAN H, SAKURAI K, et al. Voxel-based quantitative susceptibility mapping in Parkinson's disease with mild cognitive impairment[J]. Mov Disord, 2019, 34(8): 1164-1173.

[12] ATKINSON-CLEMENT C, PINTO S, EUSEBIO A,

et al. Diffusion tensor imaging in Parkinson's disease: Review and meta-analysis[J]. Neuroimage Clin, 2017, 16: 98-110.

[13] KAMAGATA K, ZALESKY A, HATANO T, et al. Gray matter abnormalities in idiopathic Parkinson's disease: evaluation by diffusional Kurtosis imaging and Neurite orientation dispersion and density imaging[J]. Hum Brain Mapp, 2017, 38(7): 3704-3722.

[14] WOLTERS, AF, VAN DE W, LEENTJES SCF, et al. Resting-state fMRI in Parkinson's disease patients with cognitive impairment: A meta-analysis[J]. Parkinsonism Relat Disord, 2019, 62: 16-27.

[15] HUANG P Y, GUAN, X J, GUO T, et al. Damaged insula network contributes to depression in Parkinson's disease [J]. Frontiers in Psychiatry, 2020, 11: 119.

[16] WANG E L, JIA Y J, YA Y, et al. Abnormal topological organization of sulcal depth-based structural covariance networks in Parkinson's disease[J]. Frontiers Aging Neuroscience, 2021, 12: 575672.

[17] HU X, QIAN L, ZHANG Y Y, et al. Topological changes in white matter connectivity network in patients with Parkinson's disease and depression[J]. Brain Imaging Behav, 2020, 14(6): 2559-2568.

[18] SREENIVASAN K, MISHRA V, BIRD C, et al. Altered functional network topology correlates with clinical

measures in very early-stage, drug-naive Parkinson's disease[J]. Parkinsonism Relat Disord, 2019, 62: 3-9.

[19] AVUCLU E, ELEN A. Evaluation of train and test performance of machine learning algorithms and Parkinson diagnosis with statistical measurements [J]. Med Biol Eng Comput, 2020, 58: 2775-2788.

[20] CIGDEM O, DEMIREL H. Performance analysis of different classification algorithmsusing different feature selection methods on Parkinson's disease detection[J]. Neurosci Methods, 2018, 309: 81-90.

[21] SOLANA-LAVALLE G, ROSAS-ROMERO R. Classification of PPMI MRI scans with voxel-based morphometry and machine learning to assist in the diagnosis of Parkinson's disease [J]. Comput Methods Programs Biomed, 2021, 198: 105793.

[22] CAO X, WANG X, XUE C, et al. A radiomics approach to predicting Parkinson's disease by incorporating whole-brain functional activity and gray matter structure [J]. Front Neurosci, 2020, 14: 751.

[23] PARK C H, LEE P H, LEE S K, et al. The diagnostic potential of multimodal neuroimaging measures in Parkinson's disease and atypical parkinsonism[J]. Brain Behav, 2020, 10(11): e01808.

第二章 经颅超声概论

经颅超声可以追溯到二十世纪七八十年代，其最初并非是用于帕金森病的检查，而是通过扫查脑桥至额顶叶区域，为该区域的血肿、脑积水、肿瘤等疾病提供相关影像学信息。随着超声技术的发展，经颅超声图像分辨率越来越高，能够通过颞窗获取中脑、丘脑等深部组织的结构图像。1995年德国Becker教授[1]等人通过对比30例帕金森病患者及30例非帕金森病患者的经颅超声图像，首次发现帕金森病患者存在中脑黑质（substantia nigra，SN）特异性强回声。自此以后，经颅超声技术飞速发展，并广泛应用到其他神经系统疾病的诊断当中。该技术与CT、MRI等影像学检查方法相比较，具有操作简单、可重复性好、价廉、无创等优点，受到越来越多的神经科医师的重视。迄今为止，经颅超声技术已得到国内外学者的认可，在2013年被欧洲神经病学会联盟纳入帕金森病诊断指南[2]，并在2016年被中华医学会纳入帕金森病的诊断标准之一[3]。

一、经颅超声参数设置

参照第九届欧洲神经超声会议（the Ninth Meeting of the European Society of Neurosonology and Cerebral Hemodynamics）制定的经颅超声在诊断神经变性疾病的检测参数，经颅超声检查使用 2.0 MHz~3.5 MHz 的相控阵探头，参数设置：穿透深度为 14 cm~16 cm，动态范围为 45 dB~55 dB，图像亮度、时间增益补偿可根据检查医师个人需要调节[4]。

二、检查过程

被检者取侧卧位，探头置于被检者左、右颞窗部位，紧贴皮肤并平行于耳眦线（眼外眦与外耳中点的连线）进行扇形扫描，以获取颅内结构的标准化检查切面。研究表明，5%~40%的被检者因颞窗透声不足，而无法通过经颅超声对其颅内相关结构进行评估[5,6]。

三、常用标准切面

1. 丘脑切面

探头置于颞窗，沿耳眦线水平向上倾斜 10°，可发现丘脑平面的定位标志——松果体,它由于钙化而表现为颅内组织最强回声。松果体前方等号样线状回声为第三脑室,丘脑位于第三脑室两侧,呈相对均质低回声;豆状核(lentiform nucleus,LN)位于丘脑前外侧,呈外宽内窄的扇形低回声;豆状核前方偏内侧为侧脑室前角。

① 第三脑室的测量。

第三脑室宽度的测量标准:测量一侧内缘至对侧内缘的垂直距离[7]。

② 豆状核的回声评估。

因正常的豆状核回声与周围脑实质回声一致,故无法从周围的脑实质中直接分辨出来,此时可通过丘脑和侧脑室前角的解剖关系推断豆状核的位置。通常情况下,可通过声窗来评估对侧豆状核的回声,因为从图像本身来讲,对侧结构显示在一个更大的扇形区域内。

豆状核回声可以分为Ⅰ~Ⅲ级(图2-1):

Ⅰ级:呈均匀分布的低回声,等同于周围脑实质回声[图2-1(a)];

Ⅱ级:呈散在点片状稍强回声[图2-1(b)];

Ⅲ级:呈斑片状强回声,明显高于周围脑实质回声[图2-1(c)]。

Ⅰ级为正常回声,≥Ⅱ级视为回声增强,此时可以通过平面测量的方法来获得豆状核强回声面积,但目前国内外尚未见相关定量判定标准[8]。

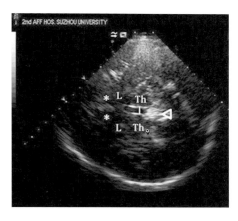

(a)

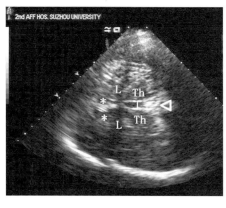

(b)

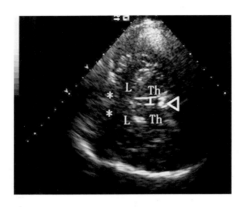

(c)

注：以颅内最强回声的松果体（三角形所示）为定位标志，第三脑室外侧后方为豆状核（L所示）。图(a)：豆状核Ⅰ级，呈均匀分布的低回声；图(b)：豆状核Ⅱ级，呈散在点片状稍强回声；图(c)：豆状核Ⅲ级，呈斑片状强回声。L：豆状核。Th：丘脑。

图 2-1 TCS 探查豆状核

2. 中脑切面

在上述丘脑切面基础上，探头向受试者足侧倾斜约 10°，可获得中脑切面。在此切面中，相对均质的蝴蝶形低回声为中脑，中央的细线样强回声为中缝核，四周环绕着强回声的基底池。

① 黑质的回声评估。

由于基底池结构对回声信号存在一定干扰，故检查过程中对黑质回声仅进行同侧评估。目前对黑质回声强度的评估方法包括半定量评估和定量评估。

半定量评估，即视觉评估，根据黑质的回声强度可分为Ⅰ-Ⅴ级（图2-2）：

Ⅰ级：黑质呈均匀分布的低回声[图2-2(a)]；

Ⅱ级：黑质内见散在点状、细线状稍强回声[图2-2(b)]；

Ⅲ级：黑质回声呈斑片状增强，低于脚间池回声[图2-2(c)]；

Ⅳ级：黑质回声呈斑片状增强，等同于脚间池回声[图2-2(d)]；

Ⅴ级：黑质回声呈斑片状增强，强于脚间池回声[图2-2(e)]；

其中黑质回声强度Ⅰ级为回声减低，Ⅱ级为正常，≥Ⅲ级为回声增强[9]。

定量评估，即面积测量，手动描绘黑质强回声轮廓，通过系统自动计算得出黑质强回声面积。当单侧黑质强回声面积<0.20 cm^2为正常；单侧黑质强回声面积0.20 cm^2~0.25 cm^2为回声中度增强；单侧黑质强回声面积≥0.25 cm^2为回声显著增强[10]。

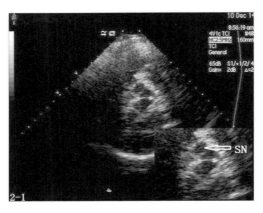

(a)

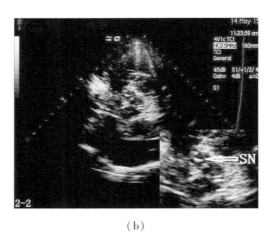

(b)

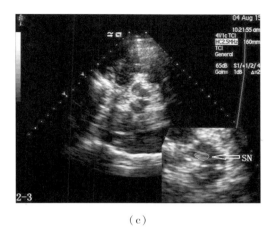

(c)

(d)

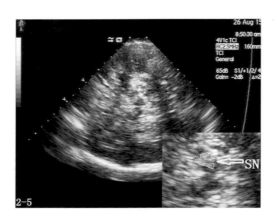

(e)

图（a）：箭头所指黑质回声强度为Ⅰ级，呈均匀分布的低回声，局部放大效果见右下角小图；图（b）：黑质回声强度Ⅱ级，黑质内见散在点状、细线状稍强回声；图（c）：黑质回声强度Ⅲ级，黑质回声呈斑片状增强，低于脚间池回声；图（d）：黑质回声强度Ⅳ级，黑质回声呈斑片状增强，等于脚间池回声；图（e）：黑质回声强度Ⅴ级，黑质回声呈斑片状增强，略高于脚间池回声。SN：黑质。

图2-2 TCS检查图及黑质回声半定量分级

因黑质、红核解剖位置较临近，对黑质进行评估时，要特别注意两者的区分。

② 中缝核的回声评估。

中缝核（midbrain raphe，BR）位于蝴蝶形中脑中央，呈连续的细线状，回声强度与红核（red

nucleus，RN）一致。由于中缝核显示较易受到被检者颞窗透声的影响，因此，如一侧颞窗探查到完整、连续的中缝核回声，即可判定为正常[11]。根据中缝核回声强度对其进行等级划分，早期研究中有三分法（1级：回声消失；2级：回声减低或中断；3级：回声正常，等同于红核）[8,11]、四分法（1级：回声消失；2级：回声中断；3级：回声减低；4级：回声正常，等同于红核）[12]，但目前共识指南建议首选二分法（0级：回声减低、中断或消失；1级：回声正常，等同于红核）[5,8,13]。

③ 大脑中动脉的测量。

在中脑平面上还可以对大脑中动脉血流进行测量。虽然经颅多普勒超声技术对大脑中动脉的血流测量研究已经十分成熟，但相对于其盲探而言，经颅超声可以通过直接显示大脑中动脉走形，提高测量部位及角度选择的准确度，具有独特的优势。

四、经颅超声的局限性及优点

经颅超声的主要局限在于：① 对受试者颞窗透声性要求较高，约10%的人群，尤其是60岁以上的女性无法获得理想图像。② 技术依赖性较强，操作医师需要经过一定的培训，否则容易导致主观性带来的误差。针对这些问题,三维容积超声、多切面自动测量等新技术正在摸索中。

经颅超声的主要优点在于操作方便快捷、费用低廉、重复性好、无创伤或辐射,经颅超声的探头同样可以用于心脏超声等检查,不会增加额外投入。适合在国内大、中型医院开展,能够为神经退行性病变的早期诊断及鉴别诊断提供一定的影像学信息,值得进一步推广和应用。

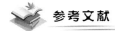

参考文献

[1] BECKER G, SEUFERT J, BOGDAHN U, et al. Degeneration of substantia nigra in chronic Parkinson's disease visualized by transcranial color-coded real-time sonography[J]. Neurology, 1995, 45(1): 182-184.

[2] BERARDELLI A, WENNING G K, ANTONINI A, et al. EFNS/MDS-ES/ENS recommendations for the diagnosis of Parkinson's disease[J]. Eur J Neurol, 2013, 20(1): 16-34.

[3] 中华医学会神经病学分会帕金森病及运动障碍学组,中国医师协会神经内科医师分会帕金森病及运动障碍专业委员会. 中国帕金森病的诊断标准(2016版)[J]. 中华神经科杂志, 2016, 49(4): 268-271.

[4] WALTER U, ŠKOLOUDÍK D. Transcranial

sonography(TCS) of brain parenchyma in movement disorders: quality standards, diagnostic applications and novel technologies [J]. Ultraschall in Med, 2014, 35: 322-331.

[5] GO C L, FRENZEL A, ROSALES R L, et al. Assessment of substantia nigra echogenicity in German and Filipino populations using a portable ultrasound system[J]. J Ultrasound Med, 2012, 31: 191-196.

[6] ŠKOLOUDIK D, WALTER U. Method and validity of transcranial sonography in movement disorders[J]. Int Rev Neurobiol, 2010, 90: 7-34.

[7] FERNANDES R D C L, BERG D. Parenchymal imaging in movement disorders[J]. Front Neurol Neurosci, 2015, 36: 71-82.

[8] WALTER U. How to measure substantia nigra hyperechogenicity in Parkinson disease: detailed guide with video[J]. J Ultrasound Med, 2013, 32(10): 1837-1843.

[9] PRESTEL J, SCHWEITZER K J, HOFER A, et al. Predictive value of transcranial sonography in the diagnosis of Parkinson's disease[J]. Mov Disord, 2006, 21(10): 1763-1765.

[10] WALTER U, BEHNKE S, EYDING J, et al. Transcranial brain parenchyma sonography in movement disorders: state of the art[J]. Ultrasound Med Biol, 2007, 33(1): 15-25.

[11] KROGIAS C, STRASSBURGER K, EYDING J, et al. Depression in patients with Huntington disease correlates with alterations of the brain stem rephe depicted by transcranial sonography[J]. Psychiatry Neurosci, 2011, 36(3): 187-194.

[12] BECKER G, BECKER T, STRUCK M, et al. Reduced echogenicity of brainstem raphe specific to unipolar depression: a transcranial color-coded real time sonography study[J]. Biol Psychiatry, 1995, 38(3): 180-184.

[13] MIJAJLOVIC M D. Transcranial sonography in depression[J]. Int Rev Neurobiol, 2010, 90: 259-272.

第三章　帕金森病经颅超声相关研究

第一节　帕金森病与经颅超声

帕金森病是最常见的神经系统退行性疾病之一，65岁以上人群发病率为0.5%~1%[1]，目前诊断主要依赖于患者的临床症状，然而当出现明显临床症状时，帕金森病患者的黑质区域50%~60%的多巴胺能神经元已丢失，纹状体系统的80%~85%多巴胺含量已减少[2]。现阶段帕金森病的治疗仅能延缓疾病病程，改善患者生活质量，并不能阻止病情的进展，所以，对帕金森病患者的早期诊断及鉴别诊断显得尤其重要。

对帕金森病的诊断，常规头颅CT、MRI缺乏特异性表现，SPECT和PET使用特殊示踪技术虽提供了较好的诊断敏感性及特异性，但是由于其装置价格昂贵、放射性物质的注射存在一定风险及辐射，难以作为临床筛查手段普及应用。

近年来，经颅超声技术通过显示帕金森病患者中脑黑质强回声进行辅助诊断，得到了国内外学者的广泛认可[3-5]。一份基于不同族群的调研发现，经颅超声诊断帕金森病的特异性达81%~92%，敏感性达78%~100%[6-9]。一项前瞻性多中心研究显示[10,11]，正常中老年人群有8%~10%伴有黑质强回声，其在未来3~5年内进展为帕金森病的概率是不伴有黑质强回声者的17.4~20.1倍。Hellwig等[12]随访了36名早期诊断不明确的帕金森病患者，结果表明经颅超声诊断早期帕金森病的特异性及敏感性分别为85%和82%。提示黑质强回声可能是帕金森病早期的一个敏感指标，这有助于我们发现帕金森病早期患者，并对健康人群进行筛查，及时发现高危人群。

关于黑质出现强回声的原因，学者们进行了深入探索。对帕金森病患者尸体解剖显示黑质强回声与其颅内异常的铁沉积相关，提示帕金森病患者黑质出现强回声可能与铁代谢功能异常有关[13]。正常情况下，大脑黑质中的大部分铁离子与颅内铁蛋白结合[14]。根据其结构，铁蛋白分为重链铁蛋白

(H-铁蛋白）和轻链铁蛋白（L-铁蛋白）。铁蛋白的轻链参与了铁在蛋白铁壳内的储存。与正常对照组相比，帕金森病患者颅内轻链铁蛋白有所下降，铁更容易从铁蛋白外排[15]。李凯等[16]研究发现，黑质回声增强的帕金森病患者相较于黑质回声正常的帕金森病患者血清铁蛋白水平更高。一项体外研究[17]认为，铁激活的小胶质细胞释放大量的神经炎症因子，增强了进展性多巴胺能神经的退行性变。

铁稳态受相关蛋白调控，包括铜蓝蛋白、铁蛋白和转铁蛋白。铜蓝蛋白将亚铁氧化为三价铁，再将含三价铁与转铁蛋白结合，这是铁转运的一种重要形式。目前研究认为，帕金森病早期阶段，颅内的铁开始重新分配其新陈代谢[18]，而总铁暂时保持不变。帕金森病患者颅内神经元的周围神经突铁含量明显升高[19]。Walter 等[20]发现 PD 患者黑质强回声与低水平的血清铁水平相关。

转铁蛋白是主要的铁转运蛋白，可以改变铁的内在化和组织储存。平衡生产脑源性转铁蛋白及其间隙可能会干扰大脑病变。Yu[21]等发现黑质强回声的帕金森病患者较黑质回声正常的帕金森病患者脑脊液铁浓度、血清转铁蛋白、血清 L-铁蛋白均有明显增高。Larumber 等[22]和一项 meta 分析[23]报告帕金森病患者外周血转铁蛋白浓度与对照组相比升高。

此外,铜蓝蛋白作为一种铁氧化酶,也参与了颅内铁水平的调节,促进细胞铁输出;遗传性铜蓝蛋白缺乏症导致铁在星形胶质细胞中堆积,并伴有类似于帕金森病的运动症状的退行性变[24]。有研究表明,血浆铜蓝蛋白基因的等位基因变异,并不会引起血浆铜蓝蛋白的完全缺失,而是改变血浆铜蓝蛋白活性[25],与此同时帕金森病患者出现黑质铁含量升高[26],这表明铁氧化酶活性减低会导致颅内铁沉积。

关于黑质强回声面积的大小与帕金森病症状的严重程度及病程,多数学者认为二者无明显相关性。一项对50名帕金森病患者近10年的随访研究发现[28],随着时间的推移,患者的临床症状逐渐加重,而黑质强回声面积并无明显改变,这说明黑质强回声是一项稳定的生物学指标,经颅超声可以作为一种较好的帕金森病辅助检查手段进行应用。

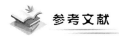

参考文献

[1] TOULOUSE A, SULLIVAN A M. Progress in Parkinson's disease—where do we stand? [J]. Prog Neurobiol, 2008, 85(4): 376-392.

[2] MILLER D B, O'CALLAGHAN J P. Biomarkers of Parkinson's disease: present and future[J]. Metabolism, 2015, 64(3 Suppl 1): S40-S46.

[3] WALTER U, SKOLOUDIK D. Transcranial sonography (TCS) of brain parenchyma in movement disorders: quality standards, diagnostic applications and novel technologies. Ultraschall in Med, 2014, 35: 322-331.

[4] 张迎春, 方军初, 盛余敬, 等. 经颅超声检查在帕金森病诊断中的应用 [J]. 中国医学影像技术, 2010, 26(12): 2255-2257.

[5] TUNC S, GRAF J, TADIC V, et al. A population-based study oncombined markers forearly Parkinson's disease [J]. Mov Disord, 2014, 30(4): 531-537.

[6] PILOTTO A, YILMAZ R, BERG D. Developments in the role of transcranial sonography for the differential diagnosis of parkinsonism[J]. Curr Neurol Neurosci Rep, 2015, 15(7): 43.

[7] BERG D, SIEFKER C, BECKER G. Echogenicity of

the substantia nigra in Parkinson's disease and its relation to clinical findings[J]. J Neurol, 2001, 248(8): 684-689.

[8] WALTER U, WITTSTOCK M, BENECKE R, et al. Substantia nigra echogenicity is normal innon-extrapyramidal cerebral disorders but increased in Parkinson's disease[J]. J Neural Transm, 2002, 109(2): 191-196.

[9] HUANG Y W, JENG J S, TSAI C F, et al. Transcranial imaging of substantia nigra hyperechogenicity in a Taiwanese cohort of Parkinson's disease[J]. Mov Disord, 2007, 22(4): 550-555.

[10] BERG D, SEPPI K, BEHNKE S, et al. Enlarged substantia nigra hyperechogenicity and risk for Parkinson's disease: a 37-month 3-center study of 1847 older persons[J]. Arch Neurol, 2011, 68(7): 932-937.

[11] BERG D, BEHNKE S, SEPPI K, et al. Enlarged hyperechogenic substantia nigra as a risk marker for Parkinson's disease[J]. Mov Disord, 2013, 28(2): 216-219.

[12] HELLWIG S, REINHARD M, AMTAGE F, et al. Transcranial sonography and [^{18}F] fluorodeoxyglucose positron emission tomography for the differential diagnosis of parkinsonism: a head-to-head comparison[J]. Eur J Neurol, 2014, 21(6): 860-866.

[13] KOSTA P, ARGYROPOULOU M, MARKOULA S, et al. MRI evaluation of the basal ganglia size and iron content in

patients with Parkinson's disease[J]. J Neurol, 2006, 253(1): 26-32.

[14] LEVI S, SANTAMBROGIO P, COZZI A, et al. The role of the L-chain in ferritin iron incorporation: studies of homo and heteropolymers[J]. J Mol Biol, 1994, 238(5): 649-654.

[15] KOZIOROWSKI D, FRIEDMAN A, AROSIO P, et al. ELISA reveals a difference in the structure of substantia nigra ferritin in Parkinson's disease and incidental Lewy body compared to control[J]. Parkinsonism Relat Disord, 2007, 13(4): 214-218.

[16] LI K, GE Y L, GU C C, et al. Substantia nigra echogenicity is associated with serum ferritin, gender and iron-related genes in Parkinson's disease[J]. Sci Rep, 2020, 10(1): 8660.

[17] ZHANG W, YAN Z F, GAO J H, et al. Role and mechanism of microglial activation in iron-induced selective and progressive dopaminergic neurodegeneration[J]. Mol Neurobiol, 2014, 49(3): 1153-1165.

[18] OWEN A D, SCHAPIRA A H, JENNER P, et al. Indices of oxidative stress in Parkinson's disease, Alzheimer's disease and dementia with Lewy bodies[J]. J Neural Transm Suppl, 1997, 51: 167-173.

[19] COSTA-MALLEN P, GATENBY C, FRIEND S, et al. Brain iron concentrations in regions of interest and relation

with serum iron levels in Parkinson disease[J]. J Neurol Sci, 2017, 378: 38-44.

[20] WALTER U, WITT R, WOLTERS A, et al. Substantia nigra echogenicity in Parkinson's disease: relation to serum iron and C-reactive protein[J]. J Neural Transm, 2012, 119: 53-57.

[21] YU S Y, CAO C J, ZUO L J, et al. Clinical features and dysfunctions of iron metabolism in Parkinson disease patients with hyper echogenicity in substantia nigra: a cross-sectional study[J]. BMC Neurol, 2018, 18(1): 9.

[22] ILUNDÁIN R L, VALLS J V F, RUEDA J J V, et al. Case-control study of markers of oxidative stress and metabolism of blood iron in Parkinson's disease[J]. Rev Esp Salud Publica, 2001, 75(1): 43-53.

[23] MARIANI S, VENTRIGLIA M, SIMONELLI I, et al. Fe and Cu do not differ in Parkinson's disease: a replication study plus meta-analysis[J]. Neurobiol Aging, 2013, 34(2): 632-633.

[24] LEVI S, FINAZZI D. Neurodegeneration with brain iron accumulation: update on pathogenic mechanisms[J]. Front Pharmacol, 2014, 5: 99.

[25] HOCHSTRASSER H, TOMIUK J, WALTER U, et al. Functional relevance of ceruloplasmin mutations in Parkinson's disease[J]. FASEB J, 2005, 19(13): 1851-1853.

[26] HOCHSTRASSER H, BAUER P, WALTER U, et al. Ceruloplasmin gene variations and substantia nigra hyperechogenicity in Parkinson disease[J]. Neurology, 2004, 63(10): 1912-1917.

[27] BEHNKE S, RUNKEL A, KASSAR H A, et al. Long-term course of substantia nigra hyperechogenicity in Parkinson's disease[J]. Mov Disord, 2013, 28(4): 455-459.

第二节 帕金森病运动症状与经颅超声

帕金森病的临床表现以锥体外系运动障碍为特征，包括运动迟缓、肌强直、静止性震颤、姿势步态障碍等。依据统一的帕金森病评分量表进行分型可分为震颤型、姿势步态异常型和其他不确定型[1,2]。

一、分类依据

根据统一的帕金森病评分量表（UPDRS-Ⅲ），帕金森病患者可以具体分为如下临床亚型：

① 姿势步态异常型（平均震颤评分/平均姿势步态异常评分<1）；

② 震颤型（平均震颤评分/平均姿势步态异常评分>1.5）；

③ 其他不确定型（1≤平均震颤评分/平均姿势步态异常评分≤1.5）。

二、病因

震颤型帕金森病患者疾病进展缓慢且预后好，而姿势步态异常型则相反，这些临床差异性产生机制至今尚未明确，目前主要研究观点如下：

① 可能与其不同的神经病理改变相关。姿势步态异常型为主型患者中红核、黑质区域存在更显著的纹状体多巴胺能神经元缺失，导致病情加剧[3]。

② 脑脊液 tau 蛋白水平升高提示细胞死亡及神经元变性。近年研究发现姿势步态异常型患者较震颤型患者脑脊液 P-tau181 水平明显升高，提示其神经元变性死亡范围更广。

③ 有研究报道发现姿势步态异常型患者情感智能障碍的病理生理基础可能与纹状体 5-羟色胺（5-HT）含量降低有关[4,5]，因此更易出现睡眠障

碍、认知障碍等非运动症状。

三、临床表现

姿势步态异常型帕金森病患者与其他两组亚表型患者相比[6]：

① 运动症状（如静止性震颤、肌强直、运动迟缓、姿势障碍等）更严重；

② 非运动症状（嗅觉减退、抑郁、焦虑、睡眠障碍等）更严重。

四、经颅超声表现

姿势步态异常型帕金森病患者与其他两组亚表型患者相比[6]：

① 黑质强回声面积更大；

② 异常黑质强回声（单侧黑质强回声面积≥0.20 cm^{2}或双侧黑质强回声面积总和/中脑面积比值≥7%）、异常中缝核回声（中缝核回声减低、中断或消失）更常见；

③ 异常豆状核回声（其回声强于脑实质回声）与第三脑室宽度（60岁前后第三脑室宽度分别超过0.7 cm、1.0 cm）之间没有明显差异。

对这些运动障碍不同临床亚表型的细化研究，

一定程度上可以解释为什么不同文献报道的帕金森病患者黑质、豆状核强回声比例不同，以及第三脑室宽度各异，因为各研究样本的病例数、性别、帕金森病病程、亚表型比例等各有不同。未来应该进一步扩大样本量，进行各临床亚型的多中心深入研究。

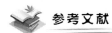
参考文献

［1］JANKOVIC J, MCDERMOTT M, CARTER J, et al. Variable expression of Parkinson's disease: a base-line analysis of the DATATOP cohort[J]. Neurology, 1990, 40(10): 1529-1534.

［2］STEBBINS G T, GOETZ C G, BURN D J, et al. How to identify tremor dominant and postural instability/gait difficulty groups with the movement disorder society unified Parkinson's disease rating scale: comparison with the unified Parkinson's disease rating scale[J]. Mov Disord, 2013, 28(5): 668-670.

［3］肖芳，张迎春，盛余敬，等．帕金森病与肌张力障碍患者经颅超声特点分析［J］．中华医学杂志，2015，95(15): 1135-1139.

［4］俞丽芳，张迎春，盛余敬，等．多系统萎缩与帕金森病患者的经颅超声研究［J］．中华老年医学杂志，

2017, 36 (1): 27-31.

[5] BECKER G, BECKER T, STRUCK M, et al. Reduced echogenicity of brainstem raphe specific to unipolar depression: a transcranial color-coded real-time sonography study [J]. Biol Psychiatry, 1995, 38(3): 180-184.

[6] SHENG A Y, ZHANG Y C, SHENG Y J, et al. Transcranial sonography image characteristics in different Parkinson's disease subtypes[J]. Neurological Sciences, 2017, 38(10): 1805-1810.

第三节 帕金森病非运动症状与经颅超声

在帕金森病的运动症状出现之前就可能有一系列的非运动症状（non-motor symptoms，NMS）出现，它们存在于整个病程中，严重影响患者的生活质量，甚至成为最困扰患者的问题。帕金森病的非运动症状种类繁多，可以分为四大类，包括神经精神障碍（抑郁、焦虑、痴呆、认知功能障碍等）、自主神经功能障碍（流涎、体位性低血压、泌尿系统障碍、勃起功能障碍、消化系统障碍、过度出汗)、睡眠障碍及感觉障碍[1]。

一、抑郁

抑郁是帕金森病患者常见的非运动症状之一,占该病患者的40%~50%[2]。相对于运动系统障碍本身而言,合并抑郁的患者预期生活质量更差[3],自杀率增高[4],给家庭和社会带来了严重的负担。但因帕金森病患者面部表情变化少,对情感描述不够清晰,导致其抑郁情绪较易被忽略。

经颅超声探查可以发现抑郁患者存在中缝核回声减低、中断或消失的特点[5],相关应用越来越多[6,7]。有报道表明50%~70%的抑郁患者存在中缝核回声异常[8,9],正常人群出现中缝核回声异常者较回声正常者发展为抑郁的风险高2.2~3.5倍[10,11]。该回声异常的机制目前尚不明确,相关研究显示,中缝核发出的5-羟色胺能神经纤维主要投射至前脑边缘及皮质[12,13],在抑郁症患者中,5-羟色胺含量明显下降,中缝核背侧核神经变性坏死明显,这可能是引起该超声声像图改变的病理学基础。

前期苏大附二院经颅超声团队研究发现,帕金森病合并抑郁患者中,脑黑质阳性率为80.0%,

中缝核阳性率为78%[14],这与国内外学者研究报道的数据相似[15],进一步证实了经颅超声技术可以探查帕金森病合并抑郁患者的黑质及中缝核回声变化。

依据汉密尔顿抑郁量表,可将抑郁依次分为轻度抑郁、中度抑郁、重度抑郁,部分文献研究表明中缝核阳性率与抑郁严重程度无关($P=0.57$)[14]。国内Zhang[16]等对40例抑郁患者经颅超声研究发现,无论是依据汉密尔顿抑郁量表还是贝克抑郁量表,中缝核回声异常与抑郁严重程度有明显相关性($P<0.05$);同时经文献调研发现,当样本量大于30时,大部分研究表明二者之间有相关性[17-20];而当样本量小于20,结果则迥异[21]。进行大样本、多种抑郁评分量表的相关性统计分析是今后研究的重要方向。

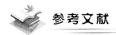

参考文献

[1] CHAUDHURI K R, YATES L, MARTINEZ-MARTIN P. The non-motor symptom complex of Parkinson's disease a comprehensive assessment is essential[J]. Curr Neurol Neurosci Rep, 2005, 5: 275-283.

[2] REIJNDERS J S, EHRT U, WEBER W, et al. A systematic review of prevalence studies of depression in Parkinson's disease[J]. Mov Disord, 2008, 23(2): 183-189.

[3] SCHRAG A. Quality of life and depression in Parkinson's disease[J]. J Neurol Sci, 2006, 248(1-2): 151-157.

[4] WHETTEN-GOLDSTEIN K, SLOAN F, KULAS E, et al. The burden of Parkinson's disease on society, family, and the individual[J]. J Am Geriatr Soc, 1997, 45(7): 844-849.

[5] BECKER G, STRUCK M, BOGDAHN U, et al. Echogenicity of the brainstem raphe in patients with major depression[J]. Psychiatry Res, 1994, 55(2): 75-84.

[6] BERG D, SEPPI K, BEHNKE S, et al. Enlarged substantia nigra hyperechogenicity and risk for Parkinson's disease: a 37-month 3-center study of 1847 older persons[J]. Arch Neurol, 2011, 68(7): 932-937.

[7] WALTER U, SKOLOUDIK D. Transcranial sonography(TCS) of brain parenchyma in movement disorders: quality standards, diagnostic applications and novel technologies [J]. Ultraschall in Med, 2014, 35(4): 322-331.

[8] MIJAJLOVIC M D. Transcranial sonography in depression[J]. Int Rev Neurobiol, 2010, 90: 259-272.

[9] WALTER U, HOEPPNER J, PRUDENTE-MORRISSEY L, et al. Parkinson's disease-like midbrain

sonography abnormalities are frequent in depressive disorders[J]. Brain, 2007, 130(7): 1799-1807.

[10] WALTER U, ŠKOLOUDÍK D, BERG D. Transcranial sonography findings related to non-motor features of Parkinson's disease[J]. Neurol Sci, 2010, 289(1-2): 123-127.

[11] STANKOVIĆ I, STEFANOVA E, ŽIROPADJA L, et al. Transcranial midbrain sonography and depressive symptoms in patients with Parkinson's disease[J]. Neurol, 2015, 262(3): 689-695.

[12] BROOKS D J, PICCINI P. Imaging in Parkinson's disease: the role of monoamines in behavior[J]. Biol Psychiatry, 2006, 59(10): 908-918.

[13] BECKER G, BERG D, LESCH K P, et al. Basal limbic system alteration in major depression: a hypothesis supported by transcranial sonography and MRI findings[J]. Neuropsycho-pharmacology, 2001, 4(1): 21-31.

[14] 王才善, 张迎春, 盛余敬, 等. 帕金森病合并抑郁患者的经颅超声神经影像学特点分析. 中华神经科杂志, 2017, 50 (7): 484-485.

[15] WALTER U, DRESSLER D, WOLTERS A, et al. Transcranial brain sonography findings in clinical subgroups of idiopathic Parkinson's disease[J]. Mov Disord, 2007, 22(1): 48-54.

[16] ZHANG Y C, HU H, LUO W F, et al. Alteration of

brainstem raphe measured by transcranial sonography in depression patients with or without Parkinson's disease [J]. Neurol Sci, 2016, 37(1): 45-50.

[17] BUDISIC M, KARLOVIC D, TRKANJEC Z, et al. Brainstem raphe lesion in patients with major depressive disorder and in patients with suicidal ideation recorded on transcranial sonography[J]. Eur Arch Psychiatry Clin Neurosci, 2010, 260(3): 203-208.

[18] CHO J W, BAIK J S, LEE M S. Mesencephalic midline change on transcranial sonography in early Parkinson's disease patients with depression[J]. Neurol Sci, 2011, 310(1-2): 50-52.

[19] WALTER U, PRUDENTE-MORRISSEY L, HERPERTZ S C, et al. Relationship of brainstem raphe echogenicity and clinical findings in depressive states [J]. Psychiatry Res, 2007, 155(1): 67-73.

[20] KROGIAS C, STRASSBURGER K, EYDING J. Depression in patients with Huntington disease correlates with alterations of the brain stem raphe depicted by transcranial sonography[J]. Psychiatry Neurosci, 2011, 36(3): 187-194.

[21] KROGIAS C, HOFFMANN K, EDYING J. Evaluation of basal ganglia, brainstem raphe and ventricles in bipolar disorder by transcranial sonography[J]. Psychiatry Res, 2011, 194(2): 190-197.

二、认知功能障碍

认知功能障碍是帕金森病患者最常见的非运动症状之一,可分为帕金森病合并轻度认知功能障碍(Parkinson's disease with mild cognitive impairment,PD-MCI)和帕金森病痴呆(Parkinson's disease with dementia,PDD)。帕金森病轻度认知功能受损是指帕金森病所致的对日常生活功能影响很小且没有进展为帕金森病痴呆的认知功能障碍综合征[1],其对帕金森病痴呆的预测风险有潜在价值,是发展为帕金森病痴呆的高危人群。帕金森病痴呆是指在确诊为原发性帕金森病的基础上,1年后出现的缓慢进展的认知功能障碍,且此认知功能障碍足以影响患者的日常生活能力。

帕金森病患者发生认知功能障碍的风险较正常老年人高 2~6 倍,但由于研究人员及临床评估标准不同,帕金森病患者中认知功能障碍的发生率在 10%~80% 不等,超过 40% 的帕金森病患者在确诊后 5 年内发生帕金森病轻度认知功能受损,最终约 80% 的帕金森病患者发展为帕金森病痴呆[2-4]。若早期发现帕金森病患者的认知功能障碍,对其预防和治疗具有重要意义。临床一般采用神经心理学量表，评估患者的认知能力、视空间和执行能力等，包含简易状态智力状态量表（mini-mental state examination，MMSE）、蒙特利尔认知评估量表（Monotreal cognitive assessment，MoCA）、画钟测试（clock-drawing test，CDT）等。帕金森病痴呆属于皮质下痴呆，以注意力、视空间能力及执行功能下降为主，其主要累及额叶皮质-纹状体环路和中脑皮层多巴胺能神经传导通路[5]。

早期研究中关于帕金森病患者运动症状的经颅超声图像特征报道较多，近年来非运动症状的相关研究也逐渐变多。帕金森病患者出现黑质强回声比例高达70%~98%，而帕金森病非痴呆患者与帕金森病痴呆患者之间，黑质强回声比例及最大面积均无显著差异，表明黑质变化指标对帕金森病患者的认知功能影响不大[6-8]。

国内外多数研究表明帕金森病患者第三脑室（third ventricle，TV）宽度与正常老年人无明显差异[9,10]，但若按照认知功能不同，可将帕金森病患者进一步划分为帕金森病认知功能正常（Parkinson's disease with normal cognition，PDNC）、帕金森病轻度认知功能受损、帕金森病痴呆，多数研究认为，帕金森病痴呆患者的第三脑室要大于帕金森病认知功能正常患者，而轻度认知功能受损患者的脑室宽度与帕金森病痴呆患者及帕金森病认知功能正常患者之间的差异尚无一致意见[7,8,11]。鉴于第三脑室增宽可能对帕金森病患者是否合并痴呆有一定鉴别意义，有报道采用 ROC 曲线进一步分析鉴别帕金森病痴呆患者与帕金森病认知功能正常患者间的第三脑室宽度界值，Dong 等[7]的研究结果表明，当第三脑室临界值为 6.8 mm 时，对区别帕金森病痴呆患者和帕金森病非痴呆患者有一定意义；Behnke 等[8]的研究进一步考虑了年龄因素，认为患者小于 70 岁时，第三脑室界值为 6 mm，而患者超过 70 岁时，第三脑室界值为 7.5 mm 则能更好地区别帕金森病痴呆患者与帕金森病认知功能正常患者。以上界值存在一定差异的原因，除年龄因素外，也可能与种族差异等因素相关。帕金森病患者的第三脑室增宽的病理可能与路易小体在新皮层和边缘系统累积，β-淀粉样蛋白等异常蛋白沉积导致皮质和皮质下萎缩相关[7,11]。

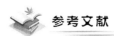

参考文献

[1] 任腾竹，聂坤，王丽娟，等. 帕金森病轻度认知

功能障碍的治疗近况[J]. 中华神经科杂志, 2017, 50(11): 876-880.

[2] BUTER T C, HOUT A V D, MATTHEWS F E, et al. Dementia and survival in Parkinson disease: a 12-year population study[J]. Neurology, 2008, 70(13): 1017-1022.

[3] HELY M A, REID W G J, ADENA M A, et al. The Sydney multicenter study of Parkinson's disease: the inevitability of dementia at 20 years[J]. Mov Disord, 2008, 23(6): 837-844.

[4] PEDERSEN K F, LARSEN J P, TYSNES O B, et al. Natural course of mild cognitive impairment in Parkinson disease: a 5-year population-based study[J]. Neurology, 2017, 88(8): 767-774.

[5] GRATWICKE J, JAHANSHAHI M, FOLTYNIE T, et al. Parkinson's disease dementia: a neural networks perspective [J]. Brain, 2015, 138(6): 1454-1476.

[6] PILOTTO A, YILMAZ R, BERG D. Developments in the role of transcranial sonography for the differential diagnosis of parkinsonism[J]. Curr Neurol Neurosci Rep, 2015, 15(7): 43.

[7] DONG Z F, WANG C S, ZHANG Y C, et al. Transcranial sonographic alterations of substantia nigra and third ventricle in Parkinson's disease with or without Dementia[J]. Chin Med J(Engl), 2017, 130(19): 2291-2295.

[8] BEHNKE S, PILOTTO A, LIEPELT-SCARFONE I,

et al. Third ventricular width assessed by transcranial ultrasound correlates with cognitive performance in Parkinson's disease[J]. Parkinsonism Relat Disord, 2019, 66: 68-73.

［9］俞丽芳，张迎春，盛余敬，等. 多系统萎缩与帕金森病患者的经颅超声研究［J］. 中华老年医学杂志，2017, 36（1）: 27-31.

［10］BOR-SENG-SHU E, PASCHOAL F M, ALMEIDA K J, et al. Transcranial brain sonography for Parkinsonian syndromes[J]. Neurosurg Sci, 2019, 63(4): 441-449.

［11］BOUWMANS A E P, LEENTJENS A F, MESS W H, et al. Abnormal echogenicity of the substantia nigra, raphe nuclei, and third-ventricle width as markers of cognitive impairment in Parkinsonian disorders: a cross-sectional study [J]. Parkinsons Dis, 2016: 1-9.

三、阻塞性睡眠呼吸暂停低通气综合征

睡眠呼吸暂停低通气综合征（sleep apnea hypopnea syndrome，SAHS）是指在睡眠过程中反复出现呼吸暂停和低通气，引起低氧血症、高碳酸血症，导致机体出现多系统损害的临床综合征[1]。睡眠呼吸暂停低通气综合征分为：阻塞性睡眠呼吸暂停低通气综合征（obstructive sleep apnea syndrome，OSAS）、中枢性睡眠呼吸暂停综合征（central sleep apnea syndrome，CSAS)、混合性睡眠呼吸暂停综合征（mixed sleep apnea syndrome，MSAS）及单纯低通气睡眠呼吸暂停综合征，其中以阻塞性睡眠呼吸暂停低通气综合征最为常见，本节主要讨论阻塞性睡眠呼吸暂停低通气综合征。

阻塞性睡眠呼吸暂停低通气综合征的特点是睡眠期间反复出现上呼吸道的部分或完全阻塞，表现为气流减少（低通气）或呼吸暂停，肺泡长期通气不畅易导致血气变化（氧脱饱和，$PaCO_2$逐渐增加），引发低氧血症、高碳酸血症、睡眠结构紊乱等。多导睡眠监测（polysomnography，PSG）是诊断阻塞性睡眠呼吸暂停低通气综合征的"金标准"。该病发病率逐年上升，据2015年统计，成年男性发病率为3%~7%，成年女性发病率为2%~5%，围绝经期女性发病率有上升趋势[2]。

阻塞性睡眠呼吸暂停低通气综合征患者长期反复的呼吸暂停可致低氧血症、高碳酸血症和脑动脉血流动力学改变，导致机体代谢、认知功能障碍，对脑血管系统的影响最为严重，睡眠呼吸暂停低通气综合征已成为脑血管疾病的独立危险因素之一，其并发生脑出血、脑梗死等的风险较健康人群明显增高。脑血管储备（cerebrovascular reserve，CVR）

是指在生理或病理因素作用下，脑血管通过微小动脉和毛细血管的代偿性收缩或扩张作用维持脑血流正常稳定的能力[3]，脑血管储备功能与阻塞性睡眠呼吸暂停低通气综合征密切相关。

经颅超声作为一项无创性体外探测颅内血管病变的影像学检查方法，主要是通过评估大脑中动脉的血流动力学变化，了解大脑动脉的弹性及顺应性，可对颅内血管病变的部位、范围、血管狭窄程度进行综合评价，为评估颅内动脉系统提供了大量的血流动力学依据。

祁风等[3]在2010年利用经颅超声技术对阻塞性睡眠呼吸暂停低通气综合征患者进行了脑血管储备功能测定，发现该类患者长期缺氧可出现颅内动脉硬化、动脉狭窄，经颅超声脑血管异常检出率高达85%。相对于对照组而言，阻塞性睡眠呼吸暂停低通气综合征组给予CO_2吸入后，脑血流速度增加值和增加率均显著降低；过度换气后，脑血流速度下降值和下降率也均显著降低。

肖淑萍等[4]通过经颅超声技术结合屏气试验评估阻塞性睡眠呼吸暂停低通气综合征患者脑血管的CO_2反应性和自动调节能力，研究表明，阻塞性睡眠呼吸暂停低通气综合征患者病情越严重，脑血流自身调节功能受损程度越大，其脑血管储备下降越明显，并发卒中风险越高。

冯浩等[5]通过比较轻度、中度、重度阻塞性睡眠呼吸暂停低通气综合征患者脑血管储备能力时发现，三组静息状态下的大脑中动脉平均速度无差别，轻度组屏气后大脑中动脉平均速度轻度下降、脑血管储备改变微小，重度组屏气后大脑中动脉平均速度显著下降、脑血管储备改变明显，说明脑血管储备改变程度随阻塞性睡眠呼吸暂停低通气综合征严重程度不同而不同，阻塞性睡眠呼吸暂停低通气综合征病情越严重，脑血管储备下降越明显。

上述变化的病理学机制可能是由于长期的睡眠呼吸暂停导致机体缺氧，刺激外周化学感受器增加体内缩血管物质的生成与释放，促使血管平滑肌增生，影响血管的收缩、舒张功能，随后并发的高碳酸血症引起脑血管收缩，使脑血流量进一步降低，最终使脑血管调节功能降低。

经颅超声技术能够对颅内动脉血流动力学进行监测，分析受检者颅内动脉是否异常（管腔狭窄、脑血管痉挛、动脉硬化、动脉供血不足等），为疾病治疗提供依据，在评估阻塞性睡眠呼吸暂停低通气综合征患者中的应用价值较高，尤其是中重度患者，可明确屏气前后大脑中动脉流速增加率，通过测定脑血管储备功能，预测阻塞性睡眠呼吸暂停低通气综合征患者脑血管并发症的发生风险，便于临床医师及时干预不良事件。

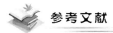

参考文献

[1] Sleep-related breathing disorders in adults: recommendations for syndrome definition and measurement techniques in clinical research.//The Report of an American Academy of Sleep Medicine Task Force[J]. Sleep, 1999, 22(5): 667-689.

[2] 阻塞性睡眠呼吸暂停低通气综合征诊治指南（基层版）写作组. 阻塞性睡眠呼吸暂停低通气综合征诊治指南（基层版）[J]. 中华全科医师杂志, 2015, 14（7）: 509-515.

[3] 祁风, 韦朝霞, 余科, 等. 经颅多普勒对睡眠呼吸暂停综合征脑血管反应能力的评价[J]. 中华全科医学, 2010, 8（1）: 11-12.

[4] 肖淑萍, 马英文, 朱海英. 阻塞性睡眠呼吸暂停低通气综合征患者脑血管自动调节潜力分析[J]. 中华神经医学杂志, 2010, 9（11）: 1137-1141.

[5] 冯浩, 张燕辉, 刘磊, 等. 经颅多普勒超声对阻塞性睡眠呼吸暂停低通气综合征脑血管反应性的评价[J].

中华老年心脑血管病杂志，2019，21（5）：511-514.

四、膀胱过度活动症

膀胱过度活动症（overactive bladder，OAB）是一种以尿频、尿急、夜尿和急迫性尿失禁为主要表现的下尿路功能障碍综合征，这些症状提示膀胱逼尿肌过度活动，各个症状可单独出现，也可多个症状同时存在。因该病各种症状易与下尿路的其他症状如尿失禁相混淆，且很多早期症状并未引起患者重视，使得流行病学相关调查研究在不同地区与国家之间差异很大。为突出下尿路症状中的储尿期症状，国际尿控协会于1999年提出了膀胱过度活动症这个概念，并于2002年对其定义做了修订[1]：在除外感染和其他病理改变的情况下，出现的尿急、伴有或不伴有急迫性尿失禁、常伴有尿频和夜尿增多的症候群，这些症状既可以单独出现，也可以多种症状同时出现。

结合我国国情，中华医学会泌尿外科分会尿控学组对膀胱过度活动症定义如下[2]：是一种以尿急症状为特征的症候群，常伴有尿频和夜尿症状，可伴有或不伴有急迫性尿失禁；在尿动力学上可能是逼尿肌过度活动，也可能是其他的膀胱尿道功能障碍。其中，尿频是指成人排尿次数日间多于8次，夜间多于2次，每次尿量小于200 mL，且膀胱排空后仍有排尿感；尿急是指一种强烈的排尿欲望，且很难被主观抑制而延迟排尿；急迫性尿失禁是指与尿急相伴随或尿急后立即出现的尿失禁现象。

文献报道称，在帕金森病进展的不同阶段，泌尿系症状的发病率为27%~80%。由于膀胱过度活动症症状与帕金森病的跌倒症状及帕金森病患者的最终预后密切相关[3]，所以为帕金森病合并膀胱过度活动症的患者提供及时有效的诊断与治疗是至关重要的。

目前帕金森病合并膀胱过度活动症症状的诊疗指南建议使用抗胆碱能药物[4]，虽然有较多研究认为抗胆碱能药物对减少成人膀胱过度活动症症状有效，但患者认知功能受损、口干、便秘等副作用较明显[5]。一项试验研究发现，抗胆碱能药物治疗可以改善尿失禁症状，但对尿频的治疗效果较差。膀胱过度活动症作为帕金森病的非运动症状之一，其发病率本身就随着年龄增长而增加，最终影响患者生活质量，严重者甚至可能导致精神心理疾病[6]。因此，寻求有效的药物治疗是当务之急。

目前膀胱过度活动症的发病机制并不明确，诊断主要依靠患者临床表现及实验室检查的排他性诊断，缺乏相对客观的生物学指标及理想的影像学诊断方法。近年来国内外学者从不同的角度对其发病机制进行了研究，其中对脑功能异常的关注度较高。研究发现，帕金森病患者泌尿系统功能障碍与神经系统损害和疾病的进展阶段相关，提示泌尿系统症状与多巴胺能神经元变性和运动障碍密切相关[7]，可能途径如下[8]：① 基底节区多巴胺能平衡丧失，导致通过脑桥排尿中心抑制膀胱收缩能力丧失，从而发生频繁的非自主性膀胱收缩；② 皮质α-突触核蛋白的病变可能影响从膀胱到皮层感觉输入的整合，导致对膀胱充盈感识别丧失，出现排尿需求的执行功能障碍。Fowler等[9]所提出的"脑-膀胱控制理论"认为，排尿过程与下丘脑、导水管周围的区域组织结构直接或间接相关。

2006年Walter等[10]应用经颅超声检查发现，与不合并膀胱过度活动症的帕金森病患者相比，合并膀胱过度活动症的帕金森病出现中缝核回声减低、中断或消失的比例较高，且中缝核回声变化评分与膀胱过度活动症的病程呈正相关。因此推测膀胱过度活动症的发病机制可能也与中缝核有关。这一发现为该病的发病机制提供了一个新思路,也为其药物研究和治疗方法提供了新的方向。

中缝核由多个亚型核团组成,包含能够分泌5-羟色胺能的神经元。5-羟色胺是一种与抑郁、暴力、睡眠障碍、食欲不振、下尿路功能障碍等各种临床症状普遍相关的神经递质[11]。有学者认为,中缝核回声的改变会伴随5-羟色胺能系统的损害[12],并且有研究证实了其形态学改变参与了抑郁症的发病机制[13]。但也有报道表明,该部位回声的变化与色氨酸功能损伤并无直接相关性[14],未来还需要进一步的多模态研究,探索中缝核回声异常在膀胱过度活动症发病机制中的作用。

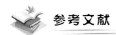

参考文献

[1] WEIN A J, ROVNER E S. Definition and epidemiology of overactive bladder[J]. Urology, 2002, 60(5 Suppl 1): 7-12.

[2] 那彦, 叶章群, 孙光. 中国泌尿外科疾病诊断治疗指南(2011版)[M]. 北京: 人民卫生出版社, 2011.

[3] VAUGHAN C P, BURGIO K L, GOODE P S, et al. Behavioral therapy for urinary symptoms in Parkinson's disease: a randomized clinical trial[J]. Neurourol Urodyn, 2019, 38

(6): 1737-1744.

[4] SEPPI K, CHANDHURI K R, COELHO M, et al. Update on treatments for nonmotor symptoms of Parkinson's disease—an evidence-based medicine review[J]. Mov Disord, 2019, 34(2): 180-198.

[5] CRISPO J A G, WILLIS A W, THIBAULT D P, et al. Associations between anticholinergic burden and adverse health outcomes in Parkinson disease[J]. PLoS One, 2016, 11(3): e0150621.

[6] VRIJENS D, DROSSAERTS J, KOEVERINGE G V, et al. Affective symptoms and the overactive bladder—a systematic review [J]. Journal of Psychosomatic Research, 2015, 78(2): 95-108.

[7] 许多, 韩顺昌, 冯娟. 帕金森病患者泌尿系统功能障碍的研究进展 [J]. 中华神经科杂志, 2019, 52 (5): 427-431.

[8] MCDONALD C, WINGE K, BURN D J. Lower urinary tract symptoms in Parkinson's disease: prevalence, aetiology and management [J]. Parkinsonism Relat Disord, 2017, 35: 8-16.

[9] FOWLER C J, GRIFFITHS D J. A decade of functional brain imaging applied to bladder control [J]. Neurourol Urodyn, 2010, 29(1): 49-55.

[10] WALTER U, DRESSLER D, WOLTERS A, et al.

Overactive bladder in Parkinson's disease: alteration of brainstem raphe detected by transcranial sonography[J]. European Journal of Neurology, 2006, 13(12): 1291-1297.

[11] LEE K S, NA Y G, DEAN-MCKINNEY T, et al. Alterations in voiding frequency and cystometry in the clomipramine induced model of endogenous depression and reversal with fluoxetine[J]. Journal of Urology, 2003, 170(5): 2067-2071.

[12] KROGIAS C, FISCHER G, MEVES S H, et al. Brainstem raphe alterations depicted by transcranial sonography do not result in serotonergic functional impairment [J]. Neuroimaging, 2013, 23(4): 477-483.

[13] ENGEL W J.Uropsychiatry[J]. Mich State Med Soc, 1964, 63: 273-277.

[14] STEWART W F, ROOYEN J B V, CUNDIFF G W, et al. Prevalence and burden of overactive bladder in the United States[J]. World Journal of Urology, 2003, 20: 327-336.

第四章　其他运动障碍性疾病与经颅超声

第一节　原发性震颤

原发性震颤（essential tremor，ET），也称特发性震颤，是一种常见的运动障碍性疾病，也是需要和帕金森病鉴别的主要疾病之一。其发病率随着年龄增加而增高[1]，但病理机制尚未明确。研究表明约60%的原发性震颤患者具有家族史[2]，此类患者体内发现有路易斯小体、浦肯野细胞磷酸化等神经退行性病变的特征，证明原发性震颤和帕金森病的发病机制在一定程度上重叠。

原发性震颤患者的主要临床表现为姿势性和运动性震颤，以上肢或头部为著，频率一般为4～16 Hz，多累及双侧，但双侧严重程度可不对称[5]。目前，其诊断主要依赖于临床表现，缺乏其他特异性的生物学诊断指标[8]。

原发性震颤和帕金森病患者在运动与非运动症状上有一定的重叠性。帕金森病患者主要表现为肢体的静止性震颤，而原发性震颤患者也可以存在静止性震颤，早期以震颤为主要症状的帕金森病患者也可以表现为动作性震颤[9,10]。就非运动症状而言，二者均可以合并抑郁、认知障碍等症状[11]。因此，对于不典型患者，通过临床症状进行鉴别存在一定困难。

经颅超声技术有助于帕金森病以及原发性震颤的鉴别诊断已经得到临床认可[12,13]。Stockner等[14]在2007年纳入了44例原发性震颤患者、100例帕金森病患者、100例健康对照者进行经颅超声检查，发现原发性震颤患者中，黑质强回声的发生率为16%，高于对照组（3%），但是低于帕金森病组（75%）。Alonso-Cánovas等[15]研究发现原发性震颤患者黑质强回声的平均面积为$0.14\ cm^2$，明显小于帕金森病组（$0.24\ cm^2$）。Richter等[16]运用经颅超声技术对31例帕金森病患者、16例原发性震颤患者、16例健康对照者的黑质进行冠状面成像，发现经颅超声技术的冠状面成像可以提高帕金森病与原发性震颤鉴别诊断的准确性（敏感性：

90.3%；特异性：96.9%）。国外经颅超声研究显示，原发性震颤患者黑质强回声发生率为0%~32%，而豆状核强回声的发生率为17.2%，其临床意义有待进一步研究[17-19]。因此，原发性震颤组黑质强回声的发生率明显低于帕金森病组，表明该指标有利于二者的鉴别诊断。

国内的相关研究也在陆续进行中。2011年，张迎春、罗蔚锋等[20]纳入100例帕金森病患者、44例原发性震颤患者、110例健康对照者进行研究，发现帕金森病组原发性震颤组及健康对照组黑质强回声的发生率分别为85.45%、13.33%、10%。王雪梅等[22]将研究对象分为原发性震颤组和原发性震颤-帕金森病组，研究发现原发性震颤组黑质强回声面积小于原发性震颤-帕金森病组。由此可见，经颅超声检查有助于对这两类患者的鉴别诊断。

相关研究表明：伴有黑质强回声的健康人群较不伴有该异常回声的健康人群而言，未来患帕金森病的风险会有所增高[23]。Kim等[24]提出，伴有黑质强回声的原发性震颤患者未来患帕金森病的风险可能也会增高。这个假设在2016年由Sprenger等[25]证实，他们纳入了54例原发性震颤患者，对其进行经颅超声检查，发现9例原发性震颤患者表现为黑质强回声，随后，他们对这9例患者进行了长达6年的随访，发现7例原发性震颤患者被诊断为帕金森病。因此，黑质强回声在原发性震颤患者中也可能是预测其帕金森病发病风险的指标。

目前，经颅超声技术对原发性震颤的价值主要在于鉴别诊断，黑质强回声在预测此类患者未来罹患帕金森病的风险上仍需更大样本的研究，多种影像学方法的横向比较研究将有助于提高诊断的准确性。

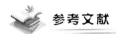
参考文献

[1] 孙虹，陈彪，孙菲，等．北京地区中老年人群原发性震颤的流行病学研究［J］．中华神经科杂志，2006，39（3）：189-192．

[2] TANNER C M, GOLDMAN S M, LYONS K E, et al. Essential tremor in twins: an assessment of genetic vs environmental determinants of etiology[J]. Neurology, 2001, 57(8): 1389-1391.

[3] DEUSCHL G, ELBLE R. Essential tremor-neurodegenerative or nondegenerative disease towards a working

definition of ET[J]. Mov Disord, 2009, 24(14): 2033-2041.

[4] LOUIS E, MAZZONI P, MA K J, et al. Essential tremor with ubiquitinated intranuclear inclusions and cerebellar degeneration[J]. Clinical Neuropathology, 2012, 31(3): 119-126.

[5] 曹红梅, 贾蕊, 曹娜, 等. 145例原发性震颤患者的临床特征分析 [J]. 西安交通大学学报（医学版）, 2016, 37（6）: 830-834, 862.

[6] 隆昱洲, 王文敏, 艾清龙. 原发性震颤患者的认知功能及抑郁情绪的研究 [J]. 中国神经精神疾病杂志, 2010, 36（1）: 23-26.

[7] CLARK L N, LOUIS E D. Essential tremor [J]. Handbook of Clinical Neurology, 2018, 147: 229-239.

[8] 中华医学会神经病学分会帕金森病及运动障碍学组. 原发性震颤的诊断和治疗指南 [J]. 中华神经科杂志, 2009, 42（8）: 571-572.

[9] HALLETT M. Parkinson's disease tremor: pathophysiology[J]. Parkinsonism Relat Disord, 2012, (18 Suppl 1): S85-86.

[10] THENGANATT M A, JANKOVIC J. The relationship between essential tremor and Parkinson's disease [J]. Parkinsonism Relat Disord, 2016, (22 Suppl 1): S162-165.

[11] LOUIS ED, WISE A, ALCALAY R N, et al. Essential tremor-Parkinson's disease: A double whammy [J].

Journal of the Neurological Sciences, 2016, 366: 47-51.

[12] 盛余敬, 张迎春, 方军初, 等. 颅脑超声对帕金森病的诊断价值 [J]. 中国医学影像技术, 2012, 28 (6): 1069-1071.

[13] 张迎春, 方军初, 盛余敬, 等. 经颅超声检查在帕金森病诊断中的应用 [J]. 中国医学影像技术, 2010, 26 (12): 2255-2257.

[14] STOCKNER H, SOJER M, MUELLER J, et al. Midbrain sonography in patients with essential tremor [J]. Mor Disord, 2007, 22(3): 414-417.

[15] ALONSO-CÁNOVAS A, LÓPEZ-SENDÓN J L, BUISÁN J, et al. Sonography for diagnosis of Parkinson disease—from theory to practice: a study on 300 participants [J]. J Ultrasound Med, 2014, 33(12): 2069-2074.

[16] RICHTER D, WOITALLA D, MUHLACK S, et al. Coronal transcranial sonography and M-mode tremor frequency determination in parkinson's disease and essential tremor [J]. J Neuroimaging, 2017, 27(5): 524-530.

[17] BÁRTOVÁ P, KRAFT O, BERNÁTEK J, et al. Transcranial sonography and ^{123}I-FP-CTP single photon emission computed tomography in movement disorders [J]. Ultrasound in Medicine & Biology, 2014, 40(10): 2365-2371.

[18] BUDISIC M, TRKANJEC Z, BOSNJAK J, et al. Distinguishing Parkinson's disease and essential tremor with

transcranial sonography [J]. Acta Neurologica Scandinavica, 2009, 119(1): 17-21.

[19] LAUĊKAITE K, ŠSURKIENE D, RASTENYTE D, et al. Specificity of transcranial sonography in parkinson spectrum disorders in comparison to degenerative cognitive syndromes[J]. BMC Neurology, 2012, 12: 12.

[20] LUO W F, ZHANG Y C, SHENG Y J, et al. Transcranial sonography on Parkinson's disease and essential tremor in a Chinese population[J]. Neurol Sci, 2012, 33(5): 1005-1009.

[21] 高红铃, 薛峥, 陶安宇, 等. 特发性震颤和帕金森病患者脑黑质高回声的相关性研究 [J]. 中华全科医师杂志, 2019, 18 (4): 365-368.

[22] 王雪梅, 曹振汤, 柳竹, 等. 特发性震颤与特发性震颤发展成帕金森病患者的临床特征比较 [J]. 中国康复理论与实践, 2018, 24 (7): 757-762.

[23] BERG D, SEPPI K, BEHNKE S, et al. Enlarged substantia nigra hyperechogenicity and risk for Parkinson disease: a 37-month 3-center study of 1847 older persons[J]. Archives of Neurology, 2011, 68(7): 932-937.

[24] KIM J S, OH Y S, KIM Y I, et al. Transcranial sonography(TCS) in Parkinson's disease (PD) and essential tremor(ET) in relation with putative premotor symptoms of PD [J]. Archives of Gerontology and Geriatrics, 2012, 54(3):

436-439.

[25] SPRENGER F S, WURSTER I, SEPPI K, et al. Substantia nigra hyperechogenicity and Parkinson's disease risk in patients with essential tremor[J]. Mov Disord, 2016, 31(4): 579-583.

第二节 多系统萎缩

多系统萎缩（multiple system atrophy，MSA）是一种散发性、病因尚未明确的神经系统变性疾病。1969年由Graham和Oppenheimers首先提出，该病男性多见，平均首次发病年龄为54~61岁，≥50岁发病率每年为（0.60~3.00）/10万人，患病率为（1.90~4.40）/10万人[1,2]。根据Gilman[3]等2008年修订的诊断标准，将多系统萎缩分型为以帕金森病样症状（运动迟缓，伴肌强直、震颤、姿势不稳等）为主的多系统萎缩-P型和以小脑症状（如步态共济失调、小脑性构音障碍、小脑性眼动障碍等）为主的多系统萎缩-C型。在西方国家，以多系统萎缩-P型多见，约占多系统萎缩的

70%~80%；在亚洲地区，以多系统萎缩-C型多见，约占多系统萎缩的60%[4-6]。该病是由于α突触核蛋白在多系统和（或）器官中异常沉积，多系统萎缩表现具有多样性，缺乏特异表现，临床诊断具有一定难度[7]。

随着影像诊断技术的发展，国内外已有较多文献报道MRI、PET、肛门括约肌肌电图等检查手段对多系统萎缩的诊断及鉴别诊断具有一定价值。多系统萎缩患者MRI主要异常征象为壳核、小脑、脑桥萎缩。T2加权像脑桥"十字形"增高影、"壳核裂隙症"为多系统萎缩相对特异的影像学表现[8,9]。FDG-PET则显示多系统萎缩患者壳核、小脑中脚及脑桥基础代谢率减低[10]。肛门括约肌肌电图通过显示肛门括约肌神经源性受损改变，有助于多系统萎缩的辅助诊断[11]。

与上述辅助诊断技术不同，经颅超声则通过显示颅内中脑及基底节核团回声改变为多系统萎缩提供神经影像学信息。相关研究显示，在多系统萎缩患者中，黑质回声多为正常，而豆状核具有明显的高回声改变[12,13]，Richter等[14]通过对15篇帕金森样综合征豆状核回声改变相关文章进行Meta分析，进一步证实了上述结果。此外，多系统萎缩患者中也表现为一定比例的第三脑室增宽[13],这些征象有助于多系统萎缩的诊断与鉴别诊断。

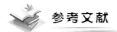
参考文献

[1] 中华医学会神经病学分会帕金森病及运动障碍学组,中国医师协会神经内科医师分会帕金森病及运动障碍专业委员会.中国帕金森病的诊断标准(2016版)[J].中华神经科杂志,2016,49(4):268-271.

[2] ERKKINEN M G, KIM M O, GESCHWIND M D. Clinical neurology and epidemiology ofthe major neurodegenerative diseases[J]. Cold Spring Harb Perspect Biol, 2018, 10(4): a033118.

[3] GILMAN S, WENNING G K, LOW P A, et al. Second consensus statement on the diagnosis of multiple system atrophy[J]. Neurology, 2008, 71(9): 670-676.

[4] JELLINGER K A. Potential clinical utility of multiple system atrophy biomarkers[J]. Expert Rev Neurother, 2017, 17(12): 1189-1208.

[5] WENNING G K, GESER F, KRISMER F, et al. The natural history of multiple system atrophy: a prospective European cohort study[J]. Lancet Neurol, 2013, 12(3): 264-274.

[6] OZAWA T, ONODERA O. Multiple system atrophy:

clinicalpathological characteristics in Japense patients[J]. Proc Jpn Acad Ser B Phys Biol Sci, 2017, 93(5): 251-258.

[7] JELLINGER K A. Neuropathology of multiple system atrophy: New thoughts about pathogenesis[J]. Mov Disord, 2014, 29(14): 1720-1741.

[8] LEE J Y, YUN J Y, SHIN C W, et al. Putaminal abnormality on 3-T magnetic resonance imaging in early parkinsonism-predominant multiple system atrophy[J]. J Neurol, 2010, 257(12): 2065-2070.

[9] 贺伟光, 范国华, 罗蔚锋, 等. 多系统萎缩和帕金森病患者的磁共振影像学分析[J]. 中华老年医学杂志, 2011, 30(3): 203-207.

[10] BROOKS D J, SEPPI K. Proposed neuroimaging criteria for the diagnosis of multiple system atrophy[J]. Mov Disord, 2009, 24(7): 949-964.

[11] YAMAMOTO T, SAKAKIBARA R, UCHIYAMA T, et al. When is Onuf's nucleus involved in multiple system atrophy? A sphincter electromyography study[J]. J Neurol Neurosurg Psychiatry, 2005, 76(12): 1645-1648.

[12] WALTER U, ŠKOLOUDIK D. Transcranial sonography(TCS) of brain parenchyma in movement disorders: quality standards, diagnostic applications and novel technologies [J]. Ultraschall Med, 2014, 35: 322-331.

[13] 俞丽芳, 张迎春, 盛余敬, 等. 多系统萎缩与帕

金森病患者的经颅超声研究［J］. 中华老年医学杂志，2017, 36（1）：27-31.

［14］RICHTER D, KATSANOS A H, SCHROEDER C, et al. Lentiform nucleus hyperechogenicity in parkinsonian syndromes: a systematic review and meta-analysis with consideration of molecular pathology［J］. Cells, 2019, 9(1): 2.

第三节 肌张力障碍

肌张力障碍（dystonia）是一种由肌肉不自主间歇或持续性收缩所导致的异常重复运动和（或）异常姿势的运动障碍性疾病，是继帕金森病及原发性震颤之后的第三大运动障碍疾病，该病致残率高，严重影响患者的生活质量。

1911年，德国神经病学家Oppenheim[1]首次提出"肌张力障碍"的命名，并以"变形性肌张力障碍"强调其肌张力变化特征。最初的肌张力障碍定义为：一种不自主、持续性肌肉收缩引起的扭曲、重复运动或姿势异常的综合征[2]。随着对该疾病相关运动现象学的不断深入了解，国际专家委员会对最初的定义进行了修订,定义已更新为:一种由肌肉不自主间歇或持续性收缩所导致的异常重复运动和(或)异常姿势的运动障碍疾病;肌张力障碍性运动一般有其模式,有扭曲动作,并且可能呈震颤性;随意动作可诱发或加重不自主动作及异常姿势,伴有"溢出"肌肉的激活[3]。

肌张力障碍最新分类主要依据临床特点和病因,用于临床诊断、判断预后和指导治疗[4]。

根据临床特点分类:

(1)根据发病年龄分类:我国第 1 版《肌张力障碍诊断与治疗指南》以 26 岁为界进行肌张力障碍分类,即早发型:≤26 岁;晚发型:>26 岁[5]。2013 年 MDS 建议将肌张力障碍参照其他神经系统疾病分类,分为婴儿(出生至 2 岁)、儿童(3~12 岁)、青少年(13~20 岁)、成年早期(21~40 岁)、成年晚期(>40 岁),以增加神经系统年龄分类的统一性。

(2)根据症状分布分类:① 局灶型:单个身体区域受累,如眼睑痉挛、口下颌肌张力障碍、书写痉挛、痉挛性构音障碍、痉挛性斜颈等。② 节段型:2 个或更多连续的身体区域受累,如 Meige 综合征等。③ 多灶型:2 个不连续或更多(连续或不连续）的身体区域受累。④ 全身型：躯干和至少 2 个其他部位受累，与以往概念不同，必须要有躯干受累而非下肢受累。⑤ 偏身型：半侧身体受累，一般都是获得性肌张力障碍，常为对侧半球损害所致。

（3）根据时间模式分类：按疾病病程不同分为稳定型和进展型。按其变异性不同分为：① 持续性型：基本持续存在，且程度接近。② 任务特异性型：仅在特定动作或任务时出现，如书写痉挛。③ 昼夜波动性型：一天内症状严重程度和表现形式存在波动，如多巴反应性肌张力障碍。④ 发作性肌张力障碍型：某一扳机事件诱发且呈自限性，突发突止。

（4）根据是否合并其他运动障碍表现分类：① 单纯性肌张力障碍：肌张力障碍是唯一的运动症状，可伴有震颤。② 复合性肌张力障碍：除肌张力障碍外，还合并其他运动障碍，如肌阵挛、帕金森症等。③ 复杂性肌张力障碍：合并其他运动障碍形式。

（5）根据是否合并其他神经系统疾病或全身受累表现分类：合并神经系统及全身受累的疾病，如 Wilson 病、脊髓小脑性共济失调（SCA）等。

根据病因分类：

（1）根据神经系统病理性分类，即根据是否存在神经系统病理改变分类，这种改变包括大体的改变、显微镜下改变或分子水平的改变。① 有神经系统退行性病变证据。② 有结构性病变证据。③ 无神经系统退行性病变或结构性病变证据。

（2）根据遗传性或获得性分类。遗传性主要指已明确相关致病基因的肌张力障碍，包括常染色体显性遗传疾病［DYT1、DYT5a、DYT6、DYT11、DYT12、脑组织铁沉积性神经变性疾病（NBIA）、齿状核红核苍白球路易体萎缩症（DRPLA）、亨廷顿病等］、常染色体隐性遗传疾病（肝豆状核变性、DYT16、DYT5b等）、X连锁隐性遗传疾病（DYT3、Lesch-Nyhan综合征、Mohr-Traneb原jaerg综合征等）、线粒体遗传等。获得性指明确存在病因的肌张力障碍，如围生期脑损伤、感染、药物、毒物、血管性、肿瘤、外伤、心因性等。

（3）根据特发性分类，即病因不明的肌张力障碍，分为散发性和家族性。

由于肌张力障碍的临床分型及疾病的发病原因复杂多样，目前尚缺乏统一的诊断标准。目前对于肌张力障碍病人的诊断，主要是结合病人的发病年龄、典型临床症状及体征、躯体受累部位、药物治疗是否有效及影像学资料等因素综合评价。

由神经系统病理性肌张力障碍的病变部位推测，原发性肌张力障碍可能是因基底神经节尤其是豆状核（lentiform nucleus，LN）发生了病理生理学改变从而导致肌肉无意识地收缩[6]。1996年，Naumann等[7]学者对肌张力障碍患者进行了经颅超声研究，结果表明75%的痉挛性斜颈患者和83%的原发性上肢肌张力障碍患者出现豆状核回声增强，1/3的面部肌张力障碍患者出现豆状核回声增强，而多巴胺反应性肌张力障碍和迟发型、运动性遗传性肌张力障碍患者中均无此表现。随后，Becker等[8]对10名痉挛性斜颈患者进行了经颅超声、MRI和^{123}I-苯甲酰胺-SPECT之间的比较研究，发现原发性肌张力障碍患者常规MRI结果均正常，而经颅超声能够较敏感地显示患者基底节区的异常，且发现70%的患者表现为豆状核回声增强。后来，Walter等[9,10]分别对特殊任务肌张力障碍患者（15名）和痉挛性构音障碍患者（14名）进行了经颅超声研究，得出豆状核回声增强的比例分别为80%、85.7%，并提出豆状核回声增强是原发性肌张力障碍的特征性表现的观点。但在此期间

Hagenah 等[11]对 84 名原发性肌张力障碍患者进行经颅超声重复研究，结果发现豆状核回声增强在原发性肌张力障碍患者中出现的比例为 57.3%，而健康对照组中出现的比例为 50%，二者之间无统计学差异，并提出豆状核回声增强并不能作为原发性肌张力障碍的一种特异性表现。

目前国内肌张力障碍的经颅超声相关研究较少，2016 年，张英、张迎春[12]等人通过对 70 名原发性局灶性肌张力障碍患者（30 名斜颈患者、30 名眼睑痉挛患者、10 名口唇异动患者）和 50 名健康对照者进行经颅超声研究，结果显示：在原发性肌张力障碍患者中，出现豆状核回声增强的整体比例（51.4%）高于正常对照组（12%）；而不同类型的原发性局灶性肌张力障碍患者之间比较，痉挛性斜颈患者豆状核回声增强的比例为 73.3%，明显高于眼睑痉挛患者（33.3%）和口唇异动患者（40.0%）；与对照组比较，痉挛性斜颈患者豆状核回声增强的比例明显高于对照组，而眼睑痉挛患者、口唇异动患者豆状核回声增强的比例与对照组之间无统计学差异，即豆状核回声增强不能作为原发性肌张力障碍患者的特征性经颅超声表现，至少不能作为眼睑痉挛和口唇异动患者的特征性表现。

鉴于以上研究存在样本量相对较小、患者病程相对较短等问题，因此，未来仍然需要长期随访以及大样本的深入研究。

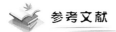

参考文献

[1] OPPENHEIM H, UBER K, DES. Dysbasia lordotica progressive, dystonia musculorum deformans-tortipelvis [J]. Neurol Zentbl, 1912, 39: 6.

[2] PAGE D, BUTLER A, JAHANSHAHI M. Quality of life in focal, segmental, and generalized dystonia [J]. Mov Disord, 2007, 22(3): 341-347.

[3] FAHN S. Concept and classification of dystonia [J]. Adv Neurol, 1988, 50: 1-8.

[4] ALBANESE A, BHATIA K, BRESSMAN S B, et al. Phenomenology and classification of dystonia: a consensus update [J]. Mov Disord, 2013, 28(7): 863-873.

[5] 中华医学会神经病学分会帕金森病及运动障碍学组. 肌张力障碍诊断与治疗指南 [J]. 中华神经科杂志, 2008, 41 (8): 570-573.

[6] BECKER G, BERG D, FRANCIAS M, et al. Evidence for disturbances of cooper metabolism in dystonia: from the image towards a new concept [J]. Neurology, 2001, 57

(12): 2290-2294.

[7] NAUMANN M, BECKER G, TOYKA K V, et al. Lenticular nucleus lesion in idiopathic dystonia detected by transcranial sonography[J]. Neurology, 1996, 47(5): 1284-1290.

[8] BECKER G, NAUMANN M, SCHEUBECK M, et al. Comparison of transcranial sonography, magnetic resonance imaging, and single photon emission computed tomography findings in idiopathic spasmodic torticollis [J]. Mov Disord, 1997, 12(1): 79-88.

[9] WALTER U, BUTTKUS F, BENECKE R, et al. Sonographic alteration of lenticular nucleus in focal task-specific dystonia of musicians [J]. Neurodegener Dis, 2012, 9(2): 99-103.

[10] WALTER U, BLITZER A, BENECKE R, et al. Sonographic detection of basal ganglia abnormalities in spasmodic dysphonia[J]. Eur J Neurol, 2014, 21(2): 349-352.

[11] HAGENAH J, KÖNIG I R, KÖTTER C, et al. Basal ganglia hyperechogenicity does not distinguish between patients with primary dystonia and healthy individuals[J]. Neurol, 2010, 258(4): 590-595.

[12] ZHANG Y, ZHANG Y C, Sheng Y J, et al. Sonographic alteration of basal ganglia in different forms of primary focal dystonia: a cross-sectional study [J]. Chinese Medical Journal, 2016, 129(8): 942-945.

第五章　经颅超声的临床实践

经颅超声（TCS）是通过颞窗获取中脑、丘脑等深部组织结构高分辨率图像的一项超声应用新技术，因该技术具有无创、无辐射、操作较为快捷、对患者依从性要求较低等优势，已经成为欧美帕金森病等运动障碍疾病患者的首选检查项目。

2009年起苏大附二院经颅超声团队在国内率先开展TCS项目，根据国外的TCS检查规范及国情，在积极加载应用超声领域各项新技术（剪切波弹性、人工智能等）的基础上，通过系统性研究，先后得到了符合我国帕金森病患者的TCS诊断标准（与2016年中国诊断指南一致），以及与其他运动障碍性疾病（原发性震颤、肌张力障碍、多系统萎缩等）的超声影像学鉴别诊断要点，并且通过深入研究，对帕金森病的不同临床亚表型、帕金森病的非运动障碍进行了进一步探索，上述系统性研究结果汇总见图5-1。

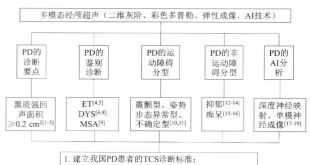

注:
PD:帕金森病;AI:人工智能;ET:原发性震颤;
DYS:肌张力障碍;MSA:多系统萎缩。

图 5-1　经颅超声系统研究图

参考文献

[1] 陈星,赵君焱,曹娴,等. 帕金森病患者经颅脑超声黑质强回声的临床特征分析 [J]. 中华神经科杂志, 2016, 49 (4): 288-293.

[2] 盛余敬,张迎春,方军初,等. 颅脑超声对帕金森病的诊断价值 [J]. 中国医学影像技术, 2012, 28 (6): 1069-1071.

[3] 张迎春,方军初,盛余敬,等. 经颅超声检查在帕金森病诊断中的应用 [J]. 中国医学影像技术, 2010, 26 (12): 2255-2257.

[4] LUO W F, ZHANG Y C, SHENG Y J, et al. Transcranial sonography on Parkinson's disease and essential tremor in a Chinese population[J]. Neurol Sci, 2012, 33(5): 1005-1009.

[5] 张迎春, 方军初, 盛余敬, 等. 帕金森病与原发性震颤患者的经颅超声研究 [J]. 中华神经科杂志, 2011, 44 (9): 590-593.

[6] ZHANG Y, ZHANG Y C, SHENG Y J, et al. Sonographic alteration of basal ganglia in different forms of primary focal dystonia: a cross-sectional study[J]. Chin Med J (Engl), 2016, 129(8): 942-945.

[7] 张英, 张迎春, 盛余敬, 等. 经颅超声诊断痉挛性斜颈 [J]. 中国医学影像技术, 2016, 32 (7): 1031-1034.

[8] 肖芳, 张迎春, 盛余敬, 等. 帕金森病与肌张力障碍患者经颅超声特点分析 [J]. 中华医学杂志, 2015, 95 (15): 1135-1139.

[9] 俞丽芳, 张迎春, 盛余敬, 等. 多系统萎缩与帕金森病患者的经颅超声研究 [J]. 中华老年医学杂志, 2017, 36 (1): 27-31.

[10] DING C W, SONG X, FU X Y, et al. Shear wave elastography characteristics of upper limb muscle in rigidity-dominant Parkinson's disease[J]. Neurological Sciences, 2021, 42(10): 4155-4162.

[11] SHENG A Y, ZHANG Y C, SHENG Y J, et al. Transcranial sonography image characteristics in different Parkinson's disease subtypes[J]. Neurol Sci, 2017, 38(10): 1805-1810.

[12] ZHANG Y C, HU H, LUO W F, et al. Alteration of brainstem raphe measured by transcranial sonography in depression patients with or without Parkinson's disease [J]. Neurol Sci, 2016, 37(1): 45-50.

[13] 傅蕴婷, 张迎春, 毛成洁, 等. 帕金森病伴骨骼肌疼痛患者中脑经颅超声回声改变研究[J]. 中华神经科杂志, 2017, 50(7): 489-495.

[14] 王才善, 张迎春, 盛余敬, 等. 帕金森病合并抑郁患者的经颅超声神经影像学特点分析[J]. 中华神经科杂志, 2017, 50(7): 484-488.

[15] 董智芬, 张迎春, 盛余敬, 等. 帕金森病与阿尔茨海默病患者的经颅超声图像分析[J]. 中国医学影像技术, 2017, 33(4): 514-517.

[16] DONG Z F, WANG C S, ZHANG Y C, et al. Transcranial sonographic alterations of substantia nigra and third ventricle in parkinson's disease with or without dementia[J]. Chin Med J(Engl), 2017, 130(19): 2291-2295.

[17] SHEN L, SHI J, DONG Y, et al. An improved deep polynomial network algorithm for transcranial sonography-based diagnosis of parkinson's disease[J]. Cognitive Computation,

2020,12(3):553-562.

[18] SHI J, XUE Z Y, DAI Y k, et al. Cascaded multi-column rvfl + classifier for single-modal neuroimaging-based diagnosis of parkinson's disease[J]. IEEE Trans Biomed Eng, 2019, 66(8): 2362-2371.

[19] GONG B M, SHI J, YING S H, et al. Neuroimaging-based diagnosis of Parkinson's disease with deep neural mapping large margin distribution machine [J]. Neurocomputing, 2018, 320: 141-149.

附　录

附录一
帕金森病的经颅超声检查操作规范流程

经颅超声作为一种超声神经系统检查新技术，已成为帕金森病患者早期诊断及鉴别诊断的主要检查方法之一。参照国外制定的 TCS 操作指南并结合我们团队前期研究经验，对 TCS 检查操作流程及标准切面概括如下。

第一步：患者取左侧卧位，探头置于患者右侧颞窗，平行于耳框线（眼角与耳廓上缘连线），识别并将探头稳定在最佳透声窗位置（图附1-1）。

第二步：获取中脑平面，其质控标准是显示中脑呈相对均质的蝴蝶样低回声，四周被高回声的脑基底池环绕，低回声区左右对称，中央为中缝核。

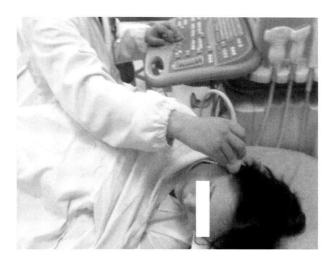

图附 1-1　检查体位图

1. 黑质

进行半定量（图附 1-2）及定量测评（详见第二章），当 SN 回声增强，需要轨迹线描绘且计算 SN 回声面积。

SN 质控标准：由于基底池结构对回声信号存在一定干扰，故对 SN 回声应进行同侧评估及面积测量[1]。此外，因 SN、红核解剖位置较临近，对 SN 进行评估时，要特别注意区分两者，切勿将红核回声误认作增强的 SN 回声。

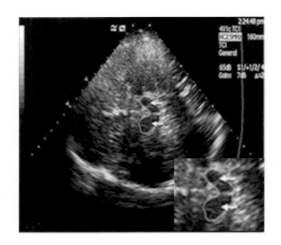

(a)

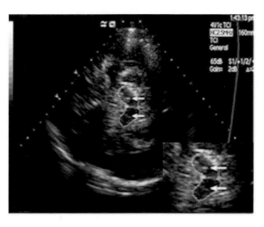

(b)

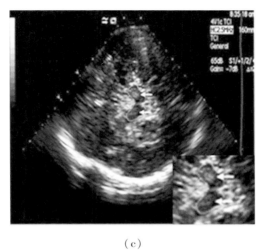

(c)

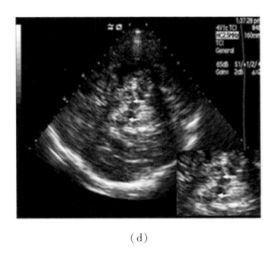

(d)

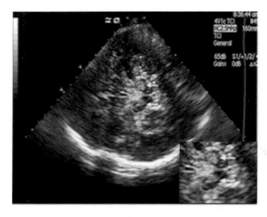

(e)

图(a)：Ⅰ级 SN 呈均匀分布的低回声；图（b）：Ⅱ级 SN 呈散在点状、细线状稍强回声；图（c）：Ⅲ级 SN 呈斑片状增强，低于脚间池回声；图（d）：Ⅳ级 SN 呈斑片状增强，等于脚间池回声；图（e）：Ⅴ级 SN 呈斑片状增强，高于脚间池回声。

图附 1-2　SN 回声半定量分级图

2. 中缝核

BR 质控标准：中脑平面基底池及红核均清晰显示[2]。正常 BR 位于蝴蝶形中脑中央，呈连续细线状，回声强度与红核一致（图附 1-3）。

BR 回声显示较易受到患者颞窗透声影响，且 BR 为纵行较长核团，因此，若在患者一侧颞窗探查到完整、连续的回声，即可判定为正常[1,3,5]。

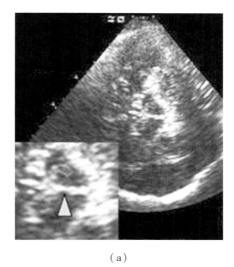

(a)

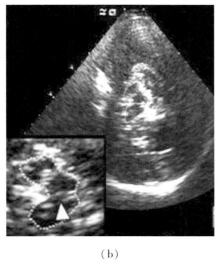

(b)

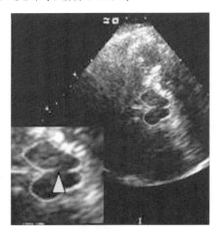

(c)

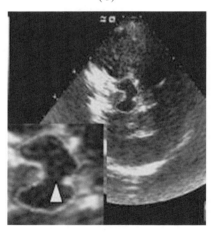

(d)

图 (a): 回声正常, 等同于 RN; 图 (b): 回声减低; 图 (c): 回声中断; 图 (d): 回声消失。

图附 1-3　中缝核回声表现图

第三步:获取丘脑平面,其质控标准是显示松果体、双侧丘脑、第三脑室及侧脑室前角。

1. 丘脑平面

在中脑平面的基础上,将探头向被检者头侧倾斜10°左右,即可见丘脑平面的定位标志——松果体(后者因钙化而表现为颅内组织最强回声,较容易辨认)。

2. 第三脑室

松果体前方两条平行细线样高回声即第三脑室(测量一侧内缘至对侧内缘的垂直距离[1]),其两侧为丘脑(图附1-4)。

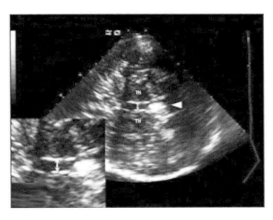

(a)

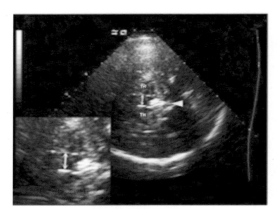

(b)

注:图(a)正常第三脑室;图(b)第三脑室增宽。

图附 1-4　第三脑室测量图

3. 豆状核

丘脑的前方可显示侧脑室前角,LN 位于丘脑和侧脑室前角之间,正常 LN 回声与周围脑实质回声一致,若 LN 回声高于周围脑实质回声,则被视为异常,即回声增强[1,4,6](图附 1-5)。

对 LN 回声应从对侧进行评估,因为对超声图像本身而言,对侧结构显示在一个更大的扇形区域内,有利于 LN 的完全显示。

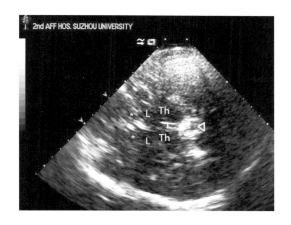

(a)

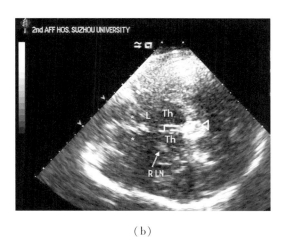

(b)

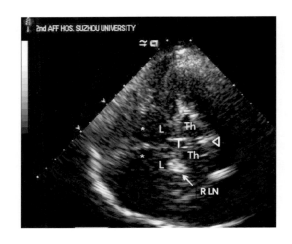

(c)

注:

图(a): Ⅰ级LN呈均匀分布的低回声, 等同于周围脑实质回声; 图(b): Ⅱ级LN呈散在点片状稍强回声; 图(c): Ⅲ级LN呈斑片状强回声, 明显高于围脑实质回声。

LN = lentiform nucleus, 豆状核, Th = thalamus, 丘脑, "△"示松果体, "＊"示侧脑室前角, "I"示第三脑室。

图附1-5 豆状核回声半定量分级图

4. 测量大脑中动脉血流及频谱质控标准

测量同侧大脑中动脉起始部[7](图附1-6)。

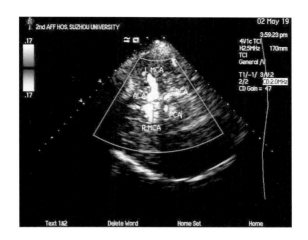

注：L MCA=左侧大脑中动脉；R MCA=右侧大脑中动脉；ACA=大脑前动脉；PCA=大脑后动脉。

图附1-6 大脑中动脉血流图

第四步：患者右侧卧位，探头置于左侧颞窗，方法步骤重复同上。

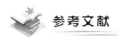

参考文献

[1] WALTER U, BEHNKE S, EYDING J, et al. Transcranial brain parenchyma sonography in movement disorders: state of the art[J]. Ultrasound Med Biol, 2007, 33(1): 15-25.

[2] WALTER U, ŠKOLOUDÍK D. Transcranial

sonography (TCS) of brain parenchyma in movement disorders: quality standards, diagnostic applications and novel technologies [J]. Ultraschall in Med, 2014, 35(4): 322-331.

[3] KROGIAS C, STRASSBURGER K, EYDING J, et al. Depression in patients with Huntington disease correlates with alterations of the brain stem rephe depicted by transcranial sonography[J]. J Psychiatry Neurosci, 2011, 36: 187-194.

[4] 肖芳, 张迎春, 盛余敬, 等. 帕金森病与肌张力障碍患者经颅超声特点分析 [J]. 中华医学杂志, 2015, 95(15): 1135-1139.

[5] ZHANG Y C, HU H, LUO W F, et al. Alteration of brainstem raphe measured by transcranial sonography in depression patients with or without Parkinson's disease [J]. Neurol Sci, 2016, 37(1): 45-50.

[6] ZHANG Y, ZHANG Y C, SHENG Y J, et al. Sonographic alteration of basal ganglia in different forms of primary focal dystonia: a cross-sectional study[J]. Chin Med J (Engl), 2016, 129(8): 942-945.

[7] DONG Z F, WANG C S, ZHANG Y C, et al. Transcranial sonographic alterations of substantia nigra and third ventricle in Parkinson's disease with or without dementia [J]. Chin Med J(Engl), 2017, 130(19): 2291-2295.

附录二
苏州大学附属第二医院 TCS 检查报告模板

TCS 探查：

第三脑室宽：

- ××cm

双侧中脑水平黑质：

- 呈线状强回声，Ⅱ级
- 右/左侧中脑水平黑质见范围约××cm²的强回声，××级，占中脑面积（cm²）的××%

中脑中线连续性：

- 好
- 回声减低
- 中断
- 消失

双侧丘脑水平豆状核：

- 未见明显异常回声
- 右/左/双侧丘脑水平豆状核回声增强

双侧大脑中动脉血流显示

➤ 正常

右侧大脑中动脉流速××cm/s；阻力指数：××

左侧大脑中动脉流速××cm/s；阻力指数：××

➤ 不清

超声提示（提出描述性诊断即可）

TCS探查结果：

未见明显异常，请结合临床。

第三脑室增宽/右/左/双侧黑质回声增强/右/左/双侧豆状核回声增强，请结合临床。

附：若患者颞窗差时，可直接描述：患者颞窗透声差，TCS效果不佳（可免费增加颈动脉超声检查）。

附录三 欧美 TCS 检查规范(2014 版)

Transcranial Sonography (TCS) of Brain Parenchyma in Movement Disorders: Quality Standards, Diagnostic Applications and Novel Technologies

Abstract

Transcranial B-mode sonography (TCS) of brain parenchyma is being increasingly used as a diagnostic tool in movement disorders. Compared to other neuroimaging modalities such as magnetic resonance imaging (MRI) and computed tomography, TCS can be performed today with portable machines and has the advantages of noninvasiveness and high resistance to movement artifacts. In distinct brain disorders TCS detects abnormalities that cannot be visualized or can only be visualized with significant effort with other imaging methods. In the field of movement disorders,

TCS has been established mainly as a tool for the early and differential diagnosis of Parkinson's disease. The postoperative position control of deep brain stimulation electrodes, especially in the subthalamic nucleus, can reliably and safely be performed with TCS. The present update review summarizes the current methodological standards and defines quality criteria of adequate TCS imaging and assessment of diagnostically relevant deep brain structures such as substantia nigra, brainstem raphe, basal ganglia and ventricles. Finally, an overview is given on recent technological advances including TCS-MRI fusion imaging and upcoming technologies of digitized image analysis aiming at a more investigator-independent assessment of deep brain structures on TCS.

Introduction

Transcranial B-mode sonography (TCS) of deep brain structures has been established as a tool for the diagnosis and monitoring of degenerative brain disorders in the past decade[1]. Several years ago, TCS could be recommended only with high-end ultrasound systems (US-S)[1,2]. Meanwhile, technological advances have enabled standard applications [assessment of the substantia nigra (SN), measurement of ventricle widths] with sufficient quality even with a portable US-S[3]. With contemporary high-end US-S, excellent image resolution of deep brain structures is achieved which can be superior to that of magnetic resonance imaging (MRI) under clinical conditions[4]. Compared to MRI and computed tomography, the advances of TCS are its high mobility, short investigation times, non-invasiveness, and low cost. Involuntary head motion in movement disorder patients can be well compensated by the investigator. Most of all, TCS detects abnormalities that are not seen, or only seen with significant effort, with other neuroimaging modalities. The present article gives an overview of the current methodological standard and defines criteria of adequate image quality for diagnostically relevant deep brain structures. In addition, recent technological advances including MRI-TCS fusion imaging and semi-automated visualization techniques are reviewed.

Method

Equipment

For TCS an optimized US-S (recommended settings, Appendix Table 3-1) equipped with a 2.0-to 3.5-MHz phased-array transducer is used. With it the highest image resolution is achieved at an image depth (distance from the transducer face) of 5-9 cm which is the so-called focal zone of the transducer[4]. Due to the physical characteristics of ultrasound beams, the image resolution in the axial direction (i.e., along the axis of ultrasound propagation) is about two-to threefold higher than in the lateral direction, usually about 0.7 mm×2 mm. This is the cause of some typical imaging artifacts (e. g., enlargement of small, highly echogenic structures in the lateral direction). Meanwhile, contemporary systems achieve a higher image resolution in the focal zone of up to 0.7 mm×1.1 mm thanks to intelligent image post-processing technologies[4]. It should be stressed that system-specific image-processing technologies influence distinct measurements such as the assessment of echogenic areas of small brain structures. That is why normal ranges especially for SN echogenic areas need to be obtained separately for each different US-S. The application of tissue harmonic imaging (THI) rather than the conventional imaging mode increases the tissue contrast and can therefore enable an easier delineation of small echogenic structures, e. g., the SN. THI however largely depends on the quality of the bone window and is not recommended as a standard tool for measurements[2].

Appendix Table 3-1 Recommended ultrasound system settings for TCS

parameter	setting
ultrasound machine	
image depth	start with 14-16 cm, adapt as needed
dynamic range	45-55 dB
post-processing function	moderate suppression of low echogenic signals
time gain compensation	adapt manually as needed or, if available, apply automated image optimization (i. e., press the referring button on the keyboard, standard with contemporary high-end ultrasound systems)

renew table

parameter	setting
image brightness	adapt manually as needed or, if available, apply automated image optimization (i.e., press the referring button on the keyboard, standard with contemporary high-end ultrasound systems)
ultrasound transducer	
density of crystals/channels	as high as possible, ideally "matrix" probe
center frequency of insonation	2.0-3.5 MHz, usually 2.5 MHz

Investigation procedures

The patient is placed in a supine position on an examination chair layer with a variably adjustable lean part. The investigation room should be darkened. The investigator sits behind the patient's head. For the usually performed transtemporal investigation, the TCS transducer is placed on the right temple near the ear and parallel to the orbitomeatal line in order to obtain a standardized axial view of intracranial structures. An important precondition for obtaining valid TCS findings is the identification and keeping of the optimum bone window for insonation. For this, the transducer is moved near the anterior helix of the ear conch to find the position with the best available visualization of brain structures and the contralateral skull bone. Once the optimum position has been found, it is kept by pressing the transducer as well as the small finger/ulnar edge of the hand firmly against the patient's head throughout the whole examination. Even if applying optimum US-S settings (Appendix Table 3-1), assessment of intracranial structures may be not or only partially possible due to an insufficient transtemporal bone window which is found in 5% ~ 40% of patients depending on age, sex and geographic origin[3-6].

➢ Quality criterion of good image quality: The contralateral skull bone is clearly visualized over its whole extension in the imaging sector.

In neurodegenerative diseases transtemporal TCS is usually carried out on standardized axial imaging planes (Appendix Fig. 3-1). For some diagnostic questions TCS is additionally performed on semi-coronal and coronal or transfrontal sagittal imaging planes, e.g. for the assessment of the corpus callosum or the localization of deep brain stimulation (DBS) electrodes[5-7]. TCS findings can be categorized into two

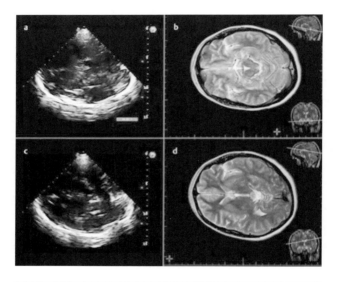

Appendix Fig. 3-1 Standard TCS axial imaging planes in movement disorders. Shown are corresponding TCS and MRI images displayed by an ultrasound system equipped with virtual navigation technology. **a** TCS image of axial transection through the brain at midbrain level. **b** MRI image corresponding to the TCS images shown in **a**. **c** TCS image of axial transection through the brain at thalamus level. **d** MRI image corresponding to the TCS images shown in **c**.

types. The first is the semi-quantitative or quantitative assessment of the echogenicity of brainstem structures (SN, red nucleus, midbrain raphe) and basal ganglia (thalamus, lenticular nucleus, head of caudate nucleus), optionally also of the cerebellum and other deep brain structures (e.g. white matter, hippocampal region). The second is the measurement of widths (optionally the cross-sectional area) of the 4th ventricle, 3rd ventricle, frontal horns of lateral ventricles and if needed the cella media.

➢ Quality criterion of adequate standard of TCS report: The report includes the rating (normal vs. abnormal) and, if obtained, the quantitative measures of echogenicity of SN, red nucleus, midbrain raphe, lenticular nucleus, caudate nucleus (and of other brain structures if investigated) as well as the widths of the 3rd ventricle and frontal horns of lateral ventricles (and of other brain structures if investigated) as well as the final interpretation of TCS findings in response to the diagnostic question.

Midbrain structures

Visualization and assessment

For many diagnostic questions in movement disorders, the visualization of midbrain structures (SN, raphe) on an axial imaging plane is of importance.

➤ Quality criterion of adequate midbrain visualization: The butterfly-shaped midbrain transection surrounded by the highly echogenic basal cisterns (cisterna ambiens, cisterna quadrigemina, cisterna suprasellaris) is completely displayed.

The SN echosignals may have a patchy, band-like or sometimes wide oval appearance (Appendix Fig. 3-2). Its appearance may slightly vary even in the same individual if using different transducer angulations or various US-S[8]. This variation is caused by the arched anatomic structure of the SN, the TCS image composition from an about 2-mm thick "slice" of the brain, the 1.5- to 3-fold higher axial than lateral TCS image resolution, and different imaging technologies of diverse US-S[6,8]. The best-validated method to grade SN echogenicity is the planimetric measurement of the SN echogenic signals on an axial plane[1,6,8-10].

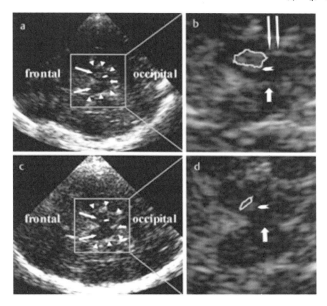

Appendix Fig. 3-2 TCS findings at axial midbrain transection. **a** In the center of the image, the butterfly-shaped, weakly echogenic midbrain is displayed which is surrounded by the highly echogenic basal cisterns (indicated by triangles). This individual exhibits a bilaterally enlarged echogenic area of substantia nigra (SN hyperechogenicity, long arrows). The lateral echosignal of ipsilateral red nucleus (arrow head) here is in conjunction with the echosignals of the SN. The short arrow indicates the typically highly echogenic aqueduct. **b** TCS image of the midbrain after zooming the image shown in a; in this panel, the echosignals of the SN are surrounded (here: enlarged echogenic area; arrow head: red nucleus; arrow: normal echogenic raphe). Note the imaging artifact originating from the basal cistern at typical position (long arrows) that should not be mistaken for SN echosignals. **c** TCS image of a subject with normal echogenic SN (long arrows; short arrow: aqueduct; arrow head: ipsilateral red nucleus) but a reduced echogenicity of midbrain raphe. **d** TCS image of the midbrain after zooming the image shown in c; in this panel, the echosignals of the SN are surrounded (here: normal echogenic area). Note the reduced echogenicity of midbrain raphe which is invisible in this example (arrow; arrow head: red nucleus).

Semiquantitative visual grading is less reliable[6,10]. Novel technologies, aiming to reduce investigator dependency, such as measuring the echointensity of the SN relative to the surrounding parenchyma, volumetry, semi-automated SN detection, or complex mathematical echo-signal analysis, have either failed or are not yet ready for clinical application[6,11-13]. Because of potential interference with echosignals originating from structures of the basal cisterns, the echogenicity of the SN is assessed only ipsilaterally to insonation. Therefore, SN TCS needs to be performed from both sides. The axial midbrain transection showing the echosignals of the ipsilateral SN in its largest extension is located by slight tilting of the probe. The clearest, most compact view of the SN echogenic signals is located by very slight probe movements. If the SN is seen very clearly, the image is frozen immediately. After choosing the optimum frame using the cine mode if necessary, the midbrain is zoomed out two-to threefold. The SN echogenic signals are surrounded manually by the cursor using the trackball, resulting in automatic calculation of the echogenic area (for video guide see[8]).

➢ Quality criterion of the adequate visualization of the SN: The echosignals of the SN are displayed at a typical anatomic location in the crus mesencephali and are well separated from the echosignals of the red nucleus and basal cisterns.

The inter-individual variation of SN echogenicity has been suggested to be caused by a variable degree of local iron accumulation and abnormal iron-protein compounds but also by gliotic changes[1,14,15]. Between the 18th and 75th year of age, the distribution of SN echogenicity can be regarded as nearly constant[16,17], even though there are reports of a moderate increase during adult life decades[18], especially after the age of 80[19]. To rate SN echogenicity in an individual as normal or increased ("hyperechogenic"), the 75th and 90th percentile of measures in the normal population are used as a reference[1], and the larger of bilaterally measured SN echogenic sizes is used for classification as follows:

➢ normal echogenic: measured area is below the 75th percentile.

➢ moderately hyperechogenic: measured area is between the 75th and the 90th percentile.

➢ markedly hyperechogenic: measured area is above the 90th percentile.

The normal ranges need to be established for each different US-S and because of some potential investigator dependency also for each different lab. For this, at least 50 healthy adults should be investigated bilaterally. Appendix Table 3-2 summarizes the cut-off values published so far for various US-S[3,10,16-18,20-25]. The evaluation of the midbrain raphe is more demanding due to a higher variability of its sonographic appearance depending on the US-S quality and settings (Appendix Table 3-1). Moreover, the assessment of the raphe is anatomically restricted to the lower midbrain with obligatory simultaneous visualization of the red nucleus. While in early reports 4 grades of echogenicity were applied (①: raphe not visible; ②: reduced or interrupted echogenicity; ③: normal, i. e., continuous line with an echogenicity similar to that of red nucleus, ④: increased echogenicity)[26], a current consensus guideline recommends the discrimination of only of two grades (normal vs. reduced echogenicity) (Appendix Fig. 3-2)[2]. Raphe echogenicity should only be classified as reduced if TCS from both sides shows reduced echogenicity under adequate imaging conditions.

Appendix Table 3-2 Reported cut-off values for the discrimination between normal echogenicity and hyperechogenicity of substantia nigra with different contemporary ultrasound systems

manufacturer/ ultrasound system	probe/ frequency [MHz]	cut-off value [cm^2]		references
		SN-h[1]	Marked SN-h[1]	
Aloka/Prosound Alpha 10	UST-52 105/2.5	≥0.19	≥0.25	Mijajlović et al.[20]
Esaote/ MyLab25 Gold	PA240/ 2.5	≥0.20	≥0.25	Go et al.[3]
Esaote/MyLab Twice	PA240/ 2.5	≥0.24	≥0.30	(own data)
General Electric/Logiq 7	3S/2.5		≥0.24	Stockner et al.[21]
General Electric/Logiq 9	3S/2.5	≥0.20		Fedotova et al.[22]

renew eable

manufacturer/ ultrasound system	probe/ frequency [MHz]	cut-off value [cm²]		references
Philips/HDI 5000 SonoCT	P2-4/2.5	≥0.20		Kim et al.[23]
Philips/HP Sonos 5500	S4/2.0~ 2.5	≥0.20	≥0.27	Mehnert et al.[17] Hagenah et al.[18]
Siemens/Acuson Antares	PX4-1/ 2.5	≥0.24	≥0.30	Van de Loo et al.[10] Glaser et al.[24]
Siemens/Sonoline Elegra	2.5PL20/ 2.6	≥0.20	≥0.25	Berg et al.[16]
Toshiba Aplio XG	PST-20CT/ 2.5	≥0.16	≥0.22	Vivo-Orti et al.[25]

SN-h = substantia nigra hyperechogenicity

1 The cut-off values for the ultrasound systems Siemens Sonoline Elegra, GE Logiq 7, Philips HP Sonos 5500 and Toshiba Aplio XG were obtained by studying large nor-mal populations. With most other TCS systems, the cut-off values were derived from receiver operating characteristic curve analysis of diagnostic discrimination between Parkinson's disease patients and healthy subjects, and/or by direct comparison of two different ultrasound systems in the same study cohort.

➢ Quality criterion of adequate assessability of the midbrain raphe: Basal cisterns, aqueduct and red nucleus are clearly displayed.

The red nucleus, located in the caudal midbrain between the raphe und SN, is typically visualized as two small stripe-like echosignals at its medial and lateral border, respectively. Sometimes its lateral echosignal cannot be discriminated from the echosignals of the SN but, if so, this usually does not relevantly interfere with measurements of the SN echogenic area. Occasionally a healthy subject exhibits marked echogenicity of the red nucleus in its full anatomical extension. This finding is rated as a hyperechogenicity even though the diagnostic meaning is unclear.

➢ Quality criterion of adequate assessability of the red nucleus: Basal cisterns, SN and midline structures (raphe, aqueduct) are clearly displayed.

Diagnostic relevance

SN hyperechogenicity is characteristically found in more than 90% of Parkinson's disease (PD) patients, does not remarkably change in the disease course and is unrelated to PD severity[1]. Marked SN hyperechogenicity is also found in about 10% of healthy adults and has been associated in them with a (subclinical) malfunction of the nigrostriatal dopaminergic system[1,16]. In a 5-year follow-up study performed in Southern Germany and Austria of 1800 subjects at ages between 50 and 70 years without PD at baseline, SN hyperechogenicity was associated with a 20-fold increased risk of developing PD[27]. However, the predictive value of this TCS finding alone is low since more than 80% of healthy subjects with SN hyperechogenicity will never develop PD during their lifetime[28]. Moreover, SN hyperechogenicity has been found with variable frequencies in a number of other neurodegenerative diseases[28]. Still, SN TCS is helpful for the discrimination of PD from essential tremor[21,29]. For the differentiation of PD from atypical Parkinsonian syndromes, SN TCS should be combined with TCS of other brain structures (Appendix Table 3-3), or with distinct clinical findings[1,30-33]. The combined presence of normal SN echogenicity and lenticular nucleus hyperechogenicity clearly discriminates atypical Parkinsonian syndromes from idiopathic PD[30,31]. In turn, the triad of SN hyperechogenicity, motor asymmetry and hyposmia is highly predictive for PD already at very early disease stages[32]. The results of several studies underpin the idea that risk scores comprising the finding of SN hyperechogenicity and other risk markers may be valuable in the prediction of subsequent PD[27,32,33]. The recently issued recommendations of the European Federation of Neurological Societies and the European Section of the Movement Disorder Society for the diagnosis of PD state that TCS is recommended (Level A) for: ① the differential diagnosis of PD from atypical Parkinsonian syndromes and secondary Parkinsonian syndromes. ② the early diagnosis of PD. ③ the detection of subjects at risk for PD[33].

Appendix Table 3-3 Typical TCS findings in normal subjects aged > 50 years and in patients with various movement disorders with a disease duration of <5 years

syndrome	hyperechogenicity of Substantia nigra	hyperechogenicity of Lenticular nucleus	dilatation of 3rd ventricle >10 mm
normal (age>50y)	(+)	+	(+)
Parkinson's disease	+++	+	(+)
Essential tremor	+	+	(+)

renew eable

syndrome	hyperechogenicity of Substantia nigra	hyperechogenicity of Lenticular nucleus	dilatation of 3rd ventricle >10 mm
MSA-P	(+)	+++	+
PSP-RS	++	+++	+++
Corticobasal degeneration	+++	+++	−
Dementia with Lewy bodies	+++	++	+
Wilson's disease	++	+++	+
Idiopathic dystonia	(+)	+++	(+)
Huntington's disease	++	++1	+

MSA-P = multiple-system atrophy, parkinsonian type; PSP-RS = progressive supranuclear palsy, Richardson syndrome. If a brain structure is assessed bilaterally, the most abnormal finding is used for classification of a patient. The symbols indicate the frequency of abnormal TCS findings in the patients investigated in our labs: − = found in no case; (+) = rarely found (<10%); + = occasionally found (10% ~ 20%); ++ = frequently found (30% ~ 50%); +++ = very frequently found (>80%).

[1] Hyperechogenicity also of the caudate nucleus is very frequently found in HD patients.

A reduced SN echogenicity (hypoechogenicity) has been demonstrated in patients with idiopathic restless legs syndrome[34,35]. SN hypoechogenicity has been proposed to be present at a sum value ≤0.20 cm^2 of bilaterally measured SN echogenic areas[35]. Its diagnostic value, however, remains to be established.

The SN represents an important landmark structure for the sonographic assessment of DBS electrode position in PD patients with DBS of the subthalamic nucleus. Optimum DBS electrode position in the subthalamic nucleus can be diagnosed on TCS if in the axial or slightly semi-axial sonogram of the midbrain the virtual tip of DBS electrode touches or "dives within" the echosignals of the SNwhich are usually hyperechogenic and therefore easily recognizable in PD patients (Appendix Fig. 3-3d)[7].

A reduced echogenicity of the midbrain raphe has been detected in about 10% of the normal population but in 50%~70% of patients with depressive disorders, and is discussed to reflect an alteration of the central serotonergic system[26,36]. Also PD and Huntington's disease patients with associated depression often exhibit this TCS feature[36-38]. The histopathological correlates and the predictive value of this finding remain to be elucidated.

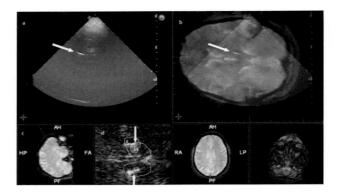

Appendix Fig. 3-3 Imaging of deep brain stimulation (DBS) electrodes on TCS. Shown are corresponding TCS and MRI images displayed by an ultrasound system equipped with virtual navigation and fusion imaging technology. a TCS image of semi-coronal transection through the brain of a patient with DBS of subthalamic nucleus. The image brightness was reduced to clearly display the DBS electrode (arrow) without reverberation artifacts. b MRI image fused with the TCS image shown in a. The DBS electrode (arrow) depicted on the TCS images projects with its tip in the subthalamic nucleus on the corresponding (pre-operatively obtained) MR image. c Panel showing the angle of the semi-coronal imaging plane applied in a, b. d Semi-coronal zoomed TCS image of the midbrain (normal image brightness; SN = substantia nigra; E = DBS electrode). The arrows indicate the virtual tips of the bilateral DBS electrodes which "dive" in the echosignals of the substantia nigra.

Cerebellum and 4th ventricle

Visualization and assessment

To approach the cerebellar imaging plane one should start at the axial midbrain plane. Then the transducer is twisted by about 45° in a semi-coronal position, with cranial movement of the anterior part of the transducer and caudal movement of the posterior part. Eventually a slight tilting of the transducer is necessary to find the optimum plane which is characterized by simultaneousdisplay of the midbrain and thalami (Appendix Fig. 3-4a). On this plane the 4th ventricle can be seen in dorsal vicinity to the midbrain. In children and young adults the 4th ventricle often cannot be recognized due to its tightness[39]. However, in elderly elderly subjects and particularly in patients with cerebellar atrophy it is usually visible. Mild cerebellar atrophy corresponds to a comma-shaped appearance, and pronounced atrophy to an oval appearance of the 4th ventricle.

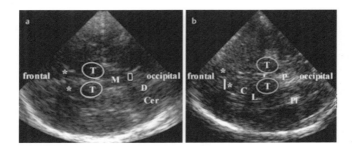

Appendix Fig. 3-4 Further standard imaging planes on TCS. **a** Cerebellar imaging plane with measurement of the 4th ventricle (rectangle). Cer = cerebellum, D = dentate nucleus, M = midbrain, T = thalamus, ∗ = frontal horn of lateral ventricle. **b** Basal-ganglia imaging plane with measurement of the 3rd ventricle (short bar) and the contralateral frontal horn (long bar). Lenticular and caudate nuclei normally are isoechogenic to surrounding brain parenchyma. C = caudate nucleus, L = lentiform nucleus, P = pineal gland, Pl = choroid plexus in the dorsal horn of lateral ventricle, T = thalamus, ∗ = frontal horn of lateral ventricle.

➢ Quality criterion of adequate assessability of the 4th ventricle and dentate nucleus: Bilateral thalami, midbrain (= reference structure), the lateral borders of the 4th ventricle and central parts of the cerebellum are clearly displayed.

There is currently no standard for the assessment of the cerebellum. Reported abnormal findings are 4th

ventricle dilatation, a coarse appearance of the cerebellar sulci, and increased echogenicity of the dentate nuclei[39,40]. Fourth-ventricle measures are the width and cross-sectional area on a semi-coronal plane. A cross-sectional area > 0.6 cm^2 can be regarded as abnormal.

Diagnostic relevance

Abnormal TCS findings of the 4th ventricle and cerebellum have been demonstrated in patients with various forms of hereditary spinocerebellar ataxia (Friedreich's ataxia, SCA-3, SCA-17)[39,40]. So far there are no reports showing a diagnostic specificity of abnormal cerebellum TCS findings, neither alone nor in combination with other TCS findings.

Basal ganglia and ventricles

Visualization and assessment

The second standard imaging plane in the assessment of movement disorders is the axial basal ganglia plane (thalamus plane). This plane is approached, if starting from the axial midbrainplane, by tilting the transducer about 20° upwards (Appendix Fig.3-1). In the case of a narrow transtemporal bone window, the transducer should be slightly shifted caudally-simultaneously with the upward tilting maneuver -in order to keep the bone window. Even if the bone window is poor, the pineal gland is mostly visible due to its calcification which therefore represents an important landmark structure of this plane. The reference structures of the axial basal ganglia plane are the bilateral, weakly echogenic thalami and the 3rd ventricle which appears as a highly echogenic double line between the thalami (Appendix Fig.3-4b). Near to the midline in a more frontal position, the frontal horns of lateral ventricles are displayed. Sometimes it is necessary to tilt the transducer slightly in a frontal direction for visualization.

➢ Quality criterion of the adequate display of the axial basal ganglia plane: Pineal gland (usually highly echogenic due to calcification), bilateral thalami (= reference structure), 3rd ventricle and contralateral frontal horn are clearly visible.

On this imaging plane the widths of the 3rd ventricle and contralateral frontal horn are measured. So far there is no consensus guideline on the location at which these measures should be obtained. While in early reports the maximum width of the 3rd ventricle was measured, most groups meanwhile prefer measuring the minimum width[2]. The width of the contralateral frontal horn is measured, as a standard in our labs, at the most frontal position at which the bilateral frontal horns are in junction (Appendix Fig. 3-4b). The measurement points are placed in a way that their conjunction line is parallel to the mid-axis of the imaging sector. Normal ranges of ventricle widths are age-dependent. In subjects under/over the age of 60, widths of >7/>10mm (3rd ventricle) and >17/>20 mm (frontal horn) are regarded as abnormal[2].

If the contralateral thalamus and the contralateral frontal horn are clearly visible, the location of the (contralateral) lenticular nucleus and caudate nucleus can be inferred from their expected anatomical position, as these basal ganglia usually are not discernible from the surrounding white matter.

Increased echogenicity, on visual assessment, of basal ganglia compared to the surrounding white matter is regarded as abnormal ("hyperechogenicity") (Appendix Fig. 3-5). Hyperechogenicity of the lenticular or caudate nucleus usually appears in a circumscribed area rather than as a diffuse change of the referring nucleus. It is important to distinguish other structures that can cause misdiagnosis of basal-ganglia hyperechogenicity due to lateral imaging artifacts. These are mainly the highly echogenic borders of the lateral ventricles, and more caudally the basal cisterns. Moreover, especially in patients with very good bone windows, reverberation artifacts originating from the highly echogenic ventricular structures (borders, choroid plexus) may mimic basal-ganglia hyperechogenicity. To avoid such misdiagnosis, it is indispensable to gain certainty about the anatomical relationship between the basal ganglia and neighboring structures potentially causing apparent hyperechogenicity by slightly tilting and twisting the transducer. Most groups assess the basal ganglia contralateral to the side of insonation (unlike SN) since the contralateral structures are displayed in a larger area in the sector-shape sonogram[2]. On the other hand, some authors prefer ipsilateral assessment of basal ganglia since they are ipsilaterally more in the focal zone of the transducer and are therefore displayed with higher image resolution. In our experience assessment of contralateral basal ganglia can be reliably performed with most US-S. However, because of higher image resolution in the focal zone, we prefer assessment of the DBS electrode position in the basal ganglia (globus pallidus internus, thalamus) ipsilaterally to the side of insonation[7]. The diagnosis of basal-ganglia hyperechogenicity is usually made visually[2]. In addition, hyperechogenic areas may be measured planimetrically, similar to measurements of SN hyperechogenicity[2,41]. Recently, the echo-intensity of basal ganglia was reliably quantified using digitized image analysis[12,42].

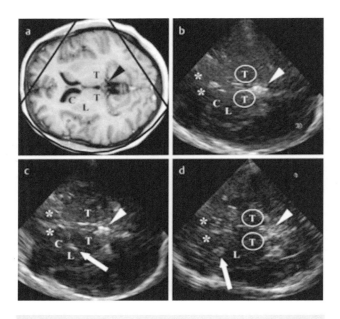

Appendix Fig. 3-5 TCS findings of basal ganglia. C = caudate nucleus, L = lenticular nucleus, T = thalamus, * = frontal horn of lateral ventricle. The triangle indicates pineal gland (highly echogenic on TCS). **a** The MR image corresponds to the sonograms in **b-d**. **b** Normal echogenicity of basal ganglia, including the lenticular nucleus. **c** Hyperechogenicity of the lenticular nucleus (arrow). **d** Hyperechogenicity of the caudate nucleus (arrow).

> Quality criterion of adequate assessability of the contralateral lenticular nucleus and caudate nucleus: Contralateral thalamus, 3rd ventricle, frontal of lateral

ventricle, and subcortical white matter (= reference structure) are clearly displayed.

Diagnostic relevance

Increasing width of the 3rd ventricle and frontal horns correlates with the degree of cognitive impairment in the normal population[43]. A pronounced dilatation of all ventricles is an instant diagnosis on TCS and indicates the presence of hydrocephalus or advanced brain atrophy[1]. Third-ventricle dilatation typically found already at early stages of progressive supranuclear palsy (Richardson syndrome) supports its discrimination from PD[31]. Hyperechogenicity of the lenticular nucleus is a characteristic finding in patients with generalized, segmental, focal and task related forms of idiopathic dystonia[41,42]. However, the specificity of this TCS finding has been challenged by one study[44], and further studies are needed to assess its diagnostic value, e. g. for the discrimination of idiopathic dystonia from psychogenic movement disorders. Lenticular nucleus hyperechogenicity is frequently detected in brain disorders with an accumulation of iron, manganese, or copper, e. g. in

Wilson's disease[14]. This finding is also present in 70% ~ 90% of patients with atypical Parkinsonian syndromes and supports, especially if combined with other TCS findings (Appendix Table 3-3), their discrimination from PD[1,30,31]. Caudate nucleus hyperechogenicity is often found in patients with Huntington's disease[38] and may support discrimination from other chorea disorders [unpublished data]. A pronounced hyperechogenicity of basal ganglia, with brightness similar to that of the pineal gland and calcified structures of the choroid plexus in the dorsal horn of the lateral ventricle, indicate calcification of the basal ganglia and may be seen as a dot—like lesion in elderly subjects but is more extended in Fahr's disease[1,45].

Novel technologies

The reliability of TCS assessment of small deep brain structures such as the SN mainly depends on two factors: ① the investigator's experience and skill, which is associated with a potential subjective bias. ② the quality of the bone window[1-6,8-10]. The influence of the latter may be reduced only slightly by lowering the insonation frequency, usually to 1.8~2.0 MHz, in the case of poor bone windows. However, the influence of the investigator dependency could potentially be overcome by applying optimized techniques for automated structure detection and digitized image analysis. Several approaches for automated SN detection and the quantification of its echogenicity have been published recently, including principal component analysisbased artificial neural networks[46], active contour segmentation algorithms[47], invariant scale blob detection[13], and 3-dimensional SN detection (volumetry) based on random forests[48]. Still, the performance of these off-line image analysis technologies is largely influenced by the quality of the TCS image primarily obtained by the investigator. So it was important to integrate a test for sufficient image quality into such software as a prerequisite for diagnostic application in the clinical routine[12]. In first clinical studies employing such a digitized image analysis tool for 2-dimensional TCS images[12], the elliptical marker highlighting the region of interest (ROI) was manually placed in the target area (SN, lenticular nucleus)[42,49]. After the placement of the ROI in the target area within the TCS image, the algorithm computes the area for each grayscale intensity I (from 0 to 255) inside the ROI area (here, size of ROI area A = 50 mm^2) (Appendix Fig.3-6). In a pilot study using this novel software[12], the automatically measured SN echogenic areas in the normal population were similar across different US-S (e. g., Esaote MyLabTwice and GE Vivid 7 Pro; r = 0.996)[49]. Moreover, manual measures of SN echogenic area obtained by highly experienced investigators correlated well with measures of digitized analysis (correlation coefficients ranging from 0.79 to 0.81)[49], as did lenticular nucleus measures (r = 0.74)[42]. The sensitivity and specificity for the diagnosis of PD based on the detection of SN hyperechogenicity by digitized image analysis were 87% and 92%, respectively[49]. In another study applying 3-dimensional quantification of SN echogenicity (volumetry), a sensitivity and specificity for the diagnosis of PD of up to 91% and 73% were reported[11].

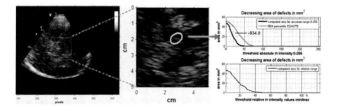

Appendix Fig. 6 Example of automated detection of the mesencephalon (window 50×50mm) within an axial sonogram of the brain at midbrain level using MATLAB-based software[12]. For automated measurement of substantia nigra echogenicity, the elliptical marker indicating the region of interest (ROI) with a size of 50 mm^2 was placed manually in the anatomical region of substantia nigra. The automated calculation of the difference between the 90th percentile cut-off value obtained from measures in normal population and the counted value in this healthy individual proved normal echogenicity of substantia nigra.

Nevertheless, the accuracy of digitized image analysis-based TCS diagnostics still depends on the investigators ability to identify and focus on the best available TCS image for visualization of a specific brain structure. Novel technologies enabling the real-time image fusion of TCS with MRI, CT or PET images, previously obtained and imported into the US-S, promise a further reduction of investigator dependency of TCS. Meanwhile, several manufacturers are marketing virtual navigation and fusion imaging applications embedded in their high-end US-S. To enable the virtual navigation on TCS-MRI fusion images, the position and orientation of the ultrasound transducer are continuously tracked by an electromagnetic system, composed of a transmitter and a small receiver, mounted on the transducer[50]. Pilot studies demonstrated a very high accuracy of fusion images, with an average cranio-caudal error of 0.5 (range, 0~0.7) cm and an average lateral shift of 0.1 (0~0.5) cm[50]. The mean time for the complete TCS examination including the fusion imaging procedure did not exceed 40 minutes. An interesting clinical application in movement disorder patients with DBS is the control of intracranial lead tip position which can be documented by the fusion of post-implantation TCS images with preoperative MRI (Appendix Fig.3-3).

All these new technologies, i.e., automated structure detection, digitized image analysis, and fusion imaging, promise a more reliable detection of brain pathologies on TCS in the future, even of brain structures that are hardly assessable visually due to their isoechogenicity to the surrounding parenchyma. This might even enable the detection of subtle changes of echogenicity over time in distinct brain structures as a correlate of disease progression.

Concluding remarks

TCS can currently be recommended in clinical practice for the assessment of ventricle widths (especially the 3rd ventricle), the early and differential diagnosis of PD, and the post-operative position control of DBS electrodes. High intra-and interrater reliability and diagnostic accuracy of planimetric SN echogenicity measurements have been demonstrated by numerous groups (for review, see[8]) which is a clear progress compared to the previous review published here in 2006[51]. The following factors impair the reliability of SN TCS and need to be excluded before diagnostic application[8]:

① the inadequate qualification of the investigator.

② the missing initial instruction and supervision of the investigator by another expert experienced in TCS in movement disorders.

③ the use of a US-S not specifically engineered and adapted for TCS.

④ inappropriate, or changing US-S settings.

⑤ the missing establishment of normal ranges of SN echogenic sizes in the referring ultrasound lab by investigation of at least 50 healthy subjects.

⑥ the variable, erroneous inclusion of highly echogenic signals of structures neighboring the SN such as the red nucleus and structures of the basal cisterns.

After excluding these sources of error, SN TCS can be learned by a physician within 2~8 weeks depending on her/his previous ultrasound experience, and is reliably performed even by adequately trained doctoral students and medical technicians[1,8]. However, the ability of reliably assessing the midbrain raphe, basal ganglia and other structures still requires more experience and supervision, at least for several months. Still, for scientific publications only TCS data should be used that were obtained by investigators who had performed and analyzed images of at least 200 patients under qualified supervision[8]. The upcoming digitized analysis and fusion imaging technologies promise a more investigator-independent assessment of deep brain structures in the near future.

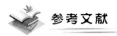

参考文献

[1] BERG D, GODAU J, WALTER U. Transcranial sonography in movement disorders[J]. Lancet Neurol, 2008, 7: 1044-1055.

[2] WALTER U, BEHNKE S, EYDING J, et al. Transcranial brain parenchyma sonography in movement disorders: state of the art[J]. Ultrasound Med Biol, 2007, 33: 15-25.

[3] GO C L, FRENZEL A, ROSALES R L, et al. Assessment of substantia nigra echogenicity in German and Filipino populations using a portable ultra-sound system[J]. J Ultrasound Med, 2012, 31: 191-196.

[4] WALTER U, KANOWSKI M, KAUFMANN J, et al. Contemporary ultrasound systems allow high-resolution transcranial imaging of small echogenic deep intracranial structures similarly as MRI: a phantom study[J]. Neuro-image, 2008, 40: 551-558.

[5] KERN R, PERREN F, KREISEL S, et al. Multiplanar transcranial ultrasound imaging: standards, landmarks and

correlation with magnetic resonance imaging[J]. Ultrasound Med Biol, 2005, 31: 311-315.

[6] SKOLOUDÍK D, WALTER U. Method and validity of transcranial sonography in movement disorders [J]. Int Rev Neurobiol, 2010, 90: 7-34.

[7] WALTER U, KIRSCH M, WITTSTOCK M, et al. Transcranial sonographic localization of deep brain stimulation electrodes is safe, reliable and predicts clinical outcome [J]. Ultrasound Med Biol, 2011, 37: 1382-1391.

[8] WALTER U. How to measure substantia nigra hyperechogenicity in Parkinson's disease: detailed guide with video[J]. J Ultrasound Med, 2013, 32: 1837-1843.

[9] ŠKOLOUDÍK D, FADRNÁT, BÁRTOVÁ P et al. Reproducibility of sonographic measurement of the substantia nigra[J]. Ultrasound Med Biol, 2007, 33: 1347-1352.

[10] VAND D L S, WALTER U, BEHNKE S, et al. Reproducibility and diagnostic accuracy of substantia nigra sonography for the diagnosis of Parkinson's disease[J]. J Neurol Neurosurg Psychiatry, 2010, 81: 1087-1092.

[11] PLATE A, AHMADI S A, PAULY O, et al. Three-dimensional sonographic examination of the midbrain for computer-aided diagnosis of movement disorders[J]. Ultrasound Med Biol, 2012, 38: 2041-2050.

[12] BLAHUTA J, SOUKUP T, ČERMÁK P, et al.

Ultrasound medical image recognition with artificial intelligence for Parkinson's disease classification [J]//BILJANOVIC P, BUTKOVIC Z, SKALA K, et al. (eds.) Proceedings of 35th International Convention on Information and Communication Technology, Electronics and Microelectronics Rijeka: Croatian Society for Information and Communication Technology. Electronics and Microelectronics-MIPRO, 2012, 958-962.

[13] CHEN L, HAGENAH J, MERTINS A. Feature analysis for Parkinson's disease detection based on transcranial sonography image[J]. Med Image Comput Comput Assist Interv, 2012, 15: 272-279.

[14] WALTER U. Transcranial sonography in brain disorders with trace metal accumulation[J]. Int Rev Neurobiol 2010, 90, 166-178.

[15] BERG D, GODAU J, RIEDERER P, et al. Microglia activation is related to substantia nigra echogenicity[J]. J Neural Transm, 2010, 117: 1287-1292.

[16] BERG D, BECKER G, ZEILER B, et al. Vulnerability of the nigrostriatal system as detected by transcranial ultrasound[J]. Neurology, 1999, 53: 1026-1031.

[17] MEHNERT S, REUTER I, SCHEPP K, et al. Transcranial sonography for diagnosis of Parkinson's disease[J]. BMC Neurol, 2010, 10: 9.

[18] HAGENAH J, KöNIG I R, SPERNER J, et al. Life-

long increase of substantia nigra hyperechogenicity in transcranial sonography[J]. Neuroimage, 2010, 51: 28-32.

[19] BEHNKE S, DOUBLE K L, DUMA S, et al. Substantia nigra echomorphology in the healthy very old: Correlation with motor slowing [J]. Neuroimage, 2007, 34: 1054-1059.

[20] MIJAJLOVI C M, DRAGASEVI C N, Stefanova E, et al. Transcranial sonography in spinocerebellar ataxia type 2[J]. J Neurol, 2008, 255: 1164-1167.

[21] STOCKNER H, SOJER M, SEPPI K, et al. Midbrain sonography in patients with essential tremor[J]. Mov Disord, 2007, 22: 414-417.

[22] FEDOTOVA E I, CHECHETKIN A O, SHADRINA M I, et al. Transcranial sonography in Parkinson's disease[J]. Zh Nevrol Psikhiatr Im S S Korsakova, 2011, 111: 49-55.

[23] KIM J Y, KIM S T, JEON S H, et al. Midbrain transcranial sonography in Korean patients with Parkinson's disease[J]. Mov Disord, 2007, 22: 1922-1926.

[24] GLASER M, WEBER U, HINRICHS H, et al. Transkranielle Sonographie des Mittelhirns mit verschiedenen Ultraschallsystemen[J]. Klin Neurophysiol, 2006, 37: 165-168.

[25] VIVO-ORTI M N, TEMBL J I, SASTRE-BATALLER I, et al. Evaluación de la sustancia negra mediante

ultrasonografía transcraneal[J]. Rev Neurol, 2013, 56: 268-274.

[26] BECKER G, BECKER T, STRUCK M, et al. Reduced echogenicity of brainstem raphe specific to unipolar depression: a transcranial color-coded real-time sonography study [J]. Biol Psychiatry, 1995, 38: 180-184.

[27] BERG D, BEHNKE S, SEPPI K, et al. Enlarged hyperechogenic substantia nigra as a risk marker for Parkinson's disease[J]. Mov Disord, 2013, 28: 216-219.

[28] WALTER U. Substantia nigra hyperechogenicity is a risk marker of Parkinson's disease: no[J]. J Neural Transm, 2011, 118: 607-612.

[29] DOEPP F, PLOTKIN M, SIEGEL L, et al. Brain parenchyma sonography and 123I-FP-CIT SPECT in Parkinson's disease and essential tremor[J]. Mov Disord, 2008, 23: 405-410.

[30] BEHNKE S, BERG D, NAUMANN M, et al. Differentiation of Parkinson's disease and atypical parkinsonian syndromes by transcranial ultrasound[J]. J Neurol Neurosurg Psychiatry, 2005, 76: 423-425.

[31] WALTER U, DRESSLER D, PROBST T, et al. Transcranial brain sonography findings in discriminating between parkinsonism and idiopathic Parkinson disease[J]. Arch Neurol, 2007, 64: 1635-1640.

[32] BUSSE K, HEILMANN R, KLEINSCHMIDT S, et al.

Value of combined midbrain sonography, olfactory and motor function assessment in the differential diagnosis of early Parkinson's disease[J]. J Neurol Neurosurg Psychiatry, 2012, 83: 441-447.

[33] BERARDELLI A, WENNING G K, ANTONINI A, et al. EFNS/MDS-ES recommendations for the diagnosis of Parkinson's disease[J]. Eur J Neurol, 2013, 20: 16-34.

[34] SCHMIDAUER C, SOJER M, SEPPI K, et al. Transcranial ultrasound shows nigral hypoechogenicity in restless legs syndrome[J]. Ann Neurol, 2005, 58: 630-634.

[35] GODAU J, SCHWEITZER K J, LIEPELT I, et al. Substantia nigra hypoechogenicity: definition and findings in restless legs syndrome[J]. Mov Disord, 2007, 22: 187-192.

[36] WALTER U, HOEPPNER J, Prudente-Morrissey L et al. Parkinson's disease-like midbrain sonography abnormalities are frequent in depressive disorders[J]. Brain, 2007, 130: 1799-1807.

[37] BERG D, SUPPRIAN T, HOFMANN E, et al. Depression in Parkinson's disease: brainstem midline alteration on transcranial sonography and magnetic resonance imaging[J]. J Neurol, 1999, 246: 1186-1193.

[38] KROGIAS C, STRASSBURGER K, EYDING J, et al. Depression in patients with Huntington disease correlates with alterations of the brain stem raphe depicted by transcranial

sonography[J]. J Psychiatry Neurosci, 2011, 36: 187-194.

[39] POSTERT T, EYDING J, BERG D, et al. Transcranial sonography in spinocerebellar ataxia type 3[J]. J Neural Transm Suppl, 2004, 68: 123-133.

[40] SYNOFZIK M, GODAU J, LINDIG T, et al. Transcranial sonography reveals cerebellar, nigral, and forebrain abnormalities in Friedreich's ataxia [J]. Neurodegener Dis, 2011, 8: 470-475.

[41] NAUMANN M, BECKER G, TOYKA K V, et al. Lenticular nucleus lesion in idiopathic dystonia detected by transcranial sonography[J]. Neurology, 1996, 47: 1284-1290.

[42] WALTER U, BLITZER A, BENECKE R, et al. Sonographic detection of basal ganglia abnormalities in spasmodic dysphonia[J]. Eur J Neurol, 2014, 21: 349-352.

[43] WOLLENWEBER F A, SCHOMBURG R, PROBST M, et al. Width of the third ventricle assessed by transcranial sonography can monitor brain atrophy in a time-and cost-effective manner-results from a longitudinal study on 500 subjects[J]. Psychiatry Res, 2011, 191: 212-216.

[44] HAGENAH J, KÖNIG IR, KÖTTER C, et al. Basal ganglia hyperechogenicity does not distinguish between patients with primary dystonia and healthy individuals[J]. J Neurol, 2011, 258: 590-595.

[45] BRÜGGEMANN N, SCHNEIDER S A, SANDER T,

et al. Distinct basal ganglia hyperechogenicity in idiopathic basal ganglia calcification[J]. Mov Disord, 2010, 25: 2661-2664.

[46] BLAHUTA J, SOUKUP T, ČERMÁK P. The image recognition of brain-stem ultrasound images with neural network based on PCA [J]//Savino M, Andria G (eds.) 2011 IEEE International Symposium on Medical Measurements and Applications (MeMeA 2011). Proceedings Bari: IEEE, 2011, 134-142.

[47] SAKALAUSKAS A, LUKOŠEVIČIUS A, LAUČKAIT E K, et al. Automated segmentation of transcranial sonographic images in the diagnostics of Parkinson's disease[J]. Ultrasonics, 2013, 53: 111-121.

[48] PAULY O, AHMADI S A, PLATE A, et al. Detection of substantia nigra echogenicities in 3D transcranial ultrasound for early diagnosis of Parkinson disease[J]. Med Image Comput Comput Assist Interv, 2012, 15: 443-450.

[49] SKOLOUDIK D, HERZIG R, BLAHUTA J, et al. Comparison of automatic and manual transcranial sonographic morphometric measurement of the substantia nigra [J]. Neurology, 2013, 80 (Meeting Abstracts 1): S39.006.

[50] FORZONI L, D'ONOFRIO S, DE B S, et al. Virtual Navigator Registration Procedure for Transcranial Application [J]//HELLMICH C, HAMZA MH, SIMSIK D (eds.) Proceedings of the IASTED International Conference Biomedical

Engineering (BioMed 2012). February 15-17, 2012 Innsbruck Austria Calgary: ACTA Press, 2012: 496-503.

[51] BERG D, BEHNKE S, WALTER U. Application of transcranial sonography in extrapyramidal disorders: updated recommendations[J]. Ultraschall in Med, 2006, 27: 12-19.

附录四 不同临床疾病经颅超声检查表现

	SN	LN	3rd V	Midbrain	Raphe
NL	nl	↑	nl	nl	↑
PD	↑ ↑	↑	nl	nl	nl or ↓
PSP-P	↑ ↑ or ↑ ↑ ↑	↑ ↑	↑	↓ ↓ ↓	nl
PSP-RS	↑	↑ ↑ ↑	↑ ↑ ↑	↓ ↓ ↓	nl
MAS	nl	↑ ↑	↑	nl	nl
CBD	↑ ↑ ↑	↑ ↑ ↑	nl	nl	nl
DLB	↑ ↑ ↑	↑ ↑	↑	nl	nl or ↓
WD	↑ ↑	↑ ↑ ↑	↑	nl or ↓	nl
ET	↑	↑	nl	nl	nl
MDD	nl	↑	nl	nl	↓ ↓
Dystonia	nl	↑ ↑ to ↑ ↑ ↑	nl	nl	nl
ALS	↑ ↑	nl	↑ ↑	nl	nl

NL：正常成人受试者；PD：帕金森病；PSP-P：以帕金森综合征为主要表型的进行性核上性麻痹；PSP-RS：以经典理查森综合征为主要表型的进行性核上性麻痹；MSA：多系统萎缩；CBD：皮质基底节变性；DLB：路易体痴呆；WD：肝豆状核变性疾病；ET：原发性震颤；MDD：以抑郁为主要表现的疾病。SN：黑质回声；LN：豆状核回声；3rd V：第三脑室宽度；中脑：中脑面积减少（横断面面积）；Rphe：中缝核回声减低；Dystonia：肌张力障碍；ALS：肌萎缩侧索硬化。

nl：发现率<10%；↑：发现率在10%~20%之间；↑↑：发现率在30%~50%之间；↑↑↑：发现率>80%；↓：介于10%~20%之间；↓↓：发现率在30%~50%之间，↓↓↓：发现率在50%~80%之间。

注：本表来源为 BERG D, GODAU J, WALTER U, et al. Transcranial sonography in movement disorders[J]. Lancet Newol, 2008, 7(11): 1044-1055.

附录五 中国帕金森病的诊断标准（2016版）

中华医学会神经病学分会帕金森病及运动障碍学组
中国医师协会神经内科医师分会帕金森病及运动障碍专业委员会

帕金森病（Parkinson's disease）是一种常见的神经系统退行性疾病，在我国65岁以上人群的患病率为1700/10万，并随年龄增长而升高，给家庭和社会带来沉重的负担[1]。该病的主要病理改变为黑质致密部多巴胺能神经元丢失和路易小体形成，其主要生化改变为纹状体区多巴胺递质降低，临床症状包括静止性震颤、肌强直、运动迟缓和姿势平衡障碍的运动症状[2]及嗅觉减退、快动眼期睡眠行为异常、便秘和抑郁等非运动症状[3]。近10年来，国内外对帕金森病的病理和病理生理、临床表现、诊断技术等方面有了更深入、全面的认识。为了更好地规范我国临床医师对帕金森病的诊断和鉴别诊断，我们在英国UK脑库帕金森病临床诊断标准的基础上,参考了国际运动障碍学会(MDS)2015 年推出的帕金森病临床诊断新标准,结合我国的实际,对我国 2006 年版的帕金森病诊断标准[4]进行了更新。

一、帕金森综合征(Parkinsonism)的诊断标准

帕金森综合征诊断的确立是诊断帕金森病的先决条件。诊断帕金森综合征基于 3 个核心运动症状,即必备运动迟缓和至少存在静止性震颤或肌强直 2 项症状的 1 项,上述症状必须是显而易见的,且与其他干扰因素无关[2]。对所有核心运动症状的检查必须按照统一帕金森病评估量表(UPDRS)中所描述的方法进行[5]。值得注意的是,MDS-UPDRS 仅能作为评估病情的手段,不能单纯地通过该量表中各项的分值来界定帕金森综合征。

二、帕金森综合征的核心运动症状

(1)运动迟缓:即运动缓慢和在持续运动中运动幅度或速度的下降(或者逐渐出现迟疑、犹豫或暂停)。该项可通过 MDS-UPDRS 中手指敲击(3.4)、手部运动(3.5)、旋前—旋后运动

(3.6)、脚趾敲击（3.7）和足部拍打（3.8）来评定。在可以出现运动迟缓症状的各个部位（包括发声、面部、步态、中轴、四肢）中，肢体运动迟缓是确立帕金森综合征诊断所必需的。

（2）肌强直：即当患者处于放松体位时，四肢及颈部主要关节的被动运动缓慢。强直特指"铅管样"抵抗，不伴有"铅管样"抵抗而单独出现的"齿轮样"强直是不满足强直的最低判定标准的。

（3）静止性震颤：即肢体处于完全静止状态时出现4~6 Hz震颤（运动起始后被抑制）。可在问诊和体检中以MDS-UPDRS中3.17和3.18为标准判断。单独的运动性和姿势性震颤（MDS-UPDRS中3.15和3.16）不满足帕金森综合征的诊断标准。

三、帕金森病的诊断

一旦患者被明确诊断存在帕金森综合征表现，可按照以下标准进行临床诊断：

（一）临床确诊的帕金森病

需要具备：（1）不存在绝对排除标准（absolute exclusion criteria）；（2）至少存在2条支持标准

（supportive criteria）；（3）没有警示征象（red flags）。

（二）临床很可能的帕金森病

需要具备：（1）不符合绝对排除标准；（2）如果出现警示征象则需要通过支持标准来抵销：如果出现1条警示征象，必须需要至少1条支持标准抵销；如果出现2条警示征象，必须需要至少2条支持标准抵销；如果出现2条以上警示征象，则诊断不能成立。

四、支持标准、绝对排除标准和警示征象

（一）支持标准

（1）患者对多巴胺能药物的治疗明确且显著有效。在初始治疗期间，患者的功能可恢复或接近至正常水平。在没有明确记录的情况下，初始治疗的显著应答可定义为以下两种情况：① 药物剂量增加时症状显著改善，剂量减少时症状显著加重。以上改变可通过客观评分（治疗后UPDRS-Ⅲ评分改善超过30%）或主观描述（由患者或看护者提供的可靠而显著的病情改变）来确定；② 存在明确且显著的开/关期症状波动，并在某种程度上包括可预测的剂末现象。

（2）出现左旋多巴诱导的异动症。

（3）临床体检观察到单个肢体的静止性震颤（既往或本次检查）。

（4）以下辅助检测阳性有助于鉴别帕金森病与非典型性帕金森综合征：存在嗅觉减退或丧失[6-14]，或头颅超声显示黑质异常高回声（>20 mm^2）[15]，或心脏间碘苄胍闪烁显像法显示心脏去交感神经支配[16-19]。

（二）绝对排除标准

出现下列任何 1 项即可排除帕金森病的诊断（但不应将有明确其他原因引起的症状算入其中，如外伤等）：

（1）存在明确的小脑性共济失调，或者小脑性眼动异常（持续的凝视诱发的眼震、巨大方波跳动、超节律扫视）。

（2）出现向下的垂直性核上性凝视麻痹，或者向下的垂直性扫视选择性减慢。

（3）在发病后 5 年内，患者被诊断为高度怀疑的行为变异型额颞叶痴呆或原发性进行性失语[20]。

（4）发病 3 年后仍局限于下肢的帕金森样症状。

（5）多巴胺受体阻滞剂或多巴胺耗竭剂治疗

诱导的帕金森综合征，其剂量和时程与药物性帕金森综合征相一致。

（6）尽管病情为中等严重程度（即根据 MDS-UPDRS，评定肌强直或运动迟缓的计分大于 2 分），但患者对高剂量（不少于 600 mg/d）左旋多巴治疗缺乏显著的治疗应答。

（7）存在明确的皮质复合感觉丧失（如在主要感觉器官完整的情况下出现皮肤书写觉和实体辨别觉损害），以及存在明确的肢体观念运动性失用或进行性失语。

（8）分子神经影像学检查突触前多巴胺能系统功能正常。

（9）存在明确可导致帕金森综合征或疑似与患者症状相关的其他疾病，或者基于全面诊断评估，由专业医师判断其可能为其他综合征，而非帕金森病[21]。

（三）警示征象

（1）发病后 5 年内出现快速进展的步态障碍，以至于需要经常使用轮椅。

（2）运动症状或体征在发病后 5 年内或 5 年以上完全不进展，除非这种病情的稳定是与治疗相关。

（3）发病后 5 年内出现球麻痹症状，表现为严重的发音困难、构音障碍或吞咽困难（须进食较软的食物，或通过鼻胃管、胃造瘘进食）。

（4）发病后 5 年内出现吸气性呼吸功能障碍，即在白天或夜间出现吸气性喘鸣或者频繁的吸气性叹息。

（5）发病后 5 年内出现严重的自主神经功能障碍，包括：① 体位性低血压[22]，即在站起后 3 min 内，收缩压下降至少 30 mmHg（1 mmHg = 0.133 kPa）或舒张压下降至少 20 mmHg，并排除脱水、药物或其他可能解释自主神经功能障碍的疾病；② 发病后 5 年内出现严重的尿潴留或尿失禁（不包括女性长期存在的低容量压力性尿失禁），且不是简单的功能性尿失禁（如不能及时如厕）。对于男性患者，尿潴留必须不是由前列腺疾病所致，且伴发勃起障碍。

（6）发病后 3 年内由于平衡障碍导致反复（＞1 次/年）跌倒。

（7）发病后 10 年内出现不成比例的颈部前倾或手足挛缩。

（8）发病后 5 年内不出现任何一种常见的非运动症状，包括嗅觉减退、睡眠障碍（睡眠维持性失眠、日间过度嗜睡、快动眼期睡眠行为障碍)、自主神经功能障碍（便秘、日间尿急、症状性体位性低血压)、精神障碍（抑郁、焦虑、幻觉)。

(9) 出现其他原因不能解释的锥体束征。

(10) 起病或病程中表现为双侧对称性的帕金森综合征症状，没有任何侧别优势，且客观体检亦未观察到明显的侧别性。

附：临床诊断标准的应用流程：

(1) 根据该标准，该患者可诊断为帕金森综合征吗？

如果答案为否，则既不能诊断为很可能的帕金森病，也不能诊断为临床确诊的帕金森病；如果答案为是，进入下一步评测。

(2) 存在任何的绝对排除标准吗？

如果答案为是，则既不能诊断为很可能的帕金森病，也不能诊断为临床确诊的帕金森病；如果答案为否，则进入下一步评测。

(3) 对出现的警示征象和支持标准进行评测，方法如下：① 记录出现警示征象的数目。② 记录支持标准的数目。③ 至少有 2 条支持标准且没有警示征象吗？如果答案为是，则患者符合临床确诊的帕金森病的诊断；如果答案为否，进入下一步评测。④ 多于 2 条警示征象吗？如果答案为是，不能诊断为很可能的帕金森病；如果答案为否，进入下一步评测。⑤ 警示征象的数目等于或少于支持标准的数目吗？如果答案为否，不能诊断为很可能的帕金森病；如果答案为是，则患者符合很可能的帕金森病的诊断。

时至今日，帕金森病仍然为一种不可治愈的疾病。但有越来越多的资料表明，对于帕金森病尽早地明确诊断并于早期进行医学、心理、社会等多方面的干预能够显著提高患者的生活质量和延长生存时间，因此对帕金森病规范地诊断和鉴别是至关重要的。另外，除了本标准所提供的基于临床信息的诊断方法外，还有包括生物学标志物、影像学、电生理、病理学等多种现行的或处于试验阶段的辅助检查手段能够协助临床医师诊断帕金森病[21]，并对其治疗方法和预后提供相应的依据，此乃不能忽视。帕金森病诊断流程图如附图 5-1 所示。

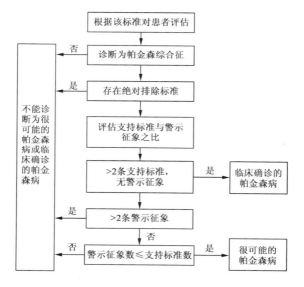

附图 5-1 帕金森病诊断流程图

参考文献

[1] ZHANG Z X, ROMAN G C, HONG Z, et al. Parkinson's disease in China: prevalence in Beijing, xi'an, and Shanghai[J]. Lancet, 2005, 365(9459): 595-597.

[2] POSTUMA R B, BERG D, STEM M, et al. MDS clinical diagnostic criteria for Parkinson's disease [J]. Mov Disord, 2015, 30(12): 1591-1601.

[3] CHAUDHURI K R, HEALY D G, SCHAPIRA A H,

et al. Non-motor symptoms of Parkinson's disease: diagnosis and management[J]. Lancet Neurol, 2006, 5(3): 235-245.

[4] 中华医学会神经病学分会帕金森病及运动障碍学组. 帕金森病的诊断 [J]. 中华神经科杂志, 2006, 39(6): 408-409.

[5] GOETZ C G, TILLEY B C, SHAFTMAN S R, et al. Movement disorder society-sponsored revision of the unified parkinson's disease rating scale (MDS-UPDRS): scale presentation and clinimetric testing results [J]. Mov Disord, 2008, 23(15): 2129-2170.

[6] SHAH M, MUHAMMED N, FINDLEY L J, et al. Olfactory tests in the diagnosis of essential tremor [J]. Parkinsonism Relat Disord, 2008, 14(7): 563-568.

[7] WENNING G K, SHEPHARD B, HAWKES C, et al. Olfactory function in atypical parkinsonian syndromes [J]. Acta Neurologica Scandinavica, 1995, 91(4): 247-250.

[8] MÜLLER A, MÜNGERSDORF M, REICHMANN H, et al. Olfactory function in Parkinsonian syndromes [J]. J Clin Neurosci, 2002, 9(5): 521-524.

[9] GOLDSTEIN D S, HOLMES C, BENTHO O, et al. Biomarkers to detect central dopamine deficiency and distinguish Parkinson disease from multiple system atrophy [J]. Parkinsonism Relat Disord, 2008, 14(8): 600-607.

[10] KATZENSCHLAGER R, ZIJLMANS J, EVANS A,

et al. Olfactory function distinguishes vascular parkinsonism from Parkinson's disease[J]. J Neurol Neurosurg Psychiatry, 2004, 75(12): 1749-1752.

[11] KIKUCHI A, BABA T, HASEGAWA T, et al. Differentiating Parkinson's disease from multiple system atrophy by [123 I]metaiodobenzylguanidine myocardial scintigraphy and olfactory test [J]. Parkinsonism Relat Disord, 2011, 17(9): 698-700.

[12] SUZUKI M, HASHIMOTO M, YOSHIOKA M, et al. The odor stick identification test for Japanese differentiates Parkinson's disease from multiple system atrophy and progressive supranuclear palsy [J]. BMC Neurol, 2011, 11(1): 157.

[13] BUSSE K, HEILMANN R, KLEINSCHMIDT S, et al. Value of combined midbrain sonography, olfactory and motor function assessment in the differential diagnosis of early Parkinson's disease[J]. J Neurol Neurosurg Psychiatry, 2012, 83(4): 441-447.

[14] RAHAYEL S, FRASNELLI J, JOUBERT S. The effect of Alzheimer's disease and Parkinson's disease on olfaction: a meta-analysis [J]. Behav Brain Res, 2012, 231 (1): 60-74.

[15] ZHOU H Y, SUN Q, TAN Y Y, et al. Substantia nigra echogenicity correlated with clinical features of Parkinson's disease [J]. Parkinsonism Relat Disord, 2016 Jan 26. Epub

ahead of print.

[16] ORIMO S, SUZUKI M, INABA A, et al. 123I-MIBG myocardial scintigraphy for differentiating Parkinson's disease from other neurodegenerative Parkinsonism: a systematic review and meta-analysis [J]. Parkinsonism Relat Disord, 2012, 18(5): 494-500.

[17] YOSHITA M, HAYASHI M, HIRAI S. Iodine 123-labeled meta-iodobenzylguanidine myocardial scintigraphy in the cases of idiopathic Parkinson's disease, multiple system atrophy, and progressive supranuclear palsy [J]. Rinsho Shinkeigaku, 1997, 37(6): 476-482.

[18] SHIN D H, LEE PH, BANG O Y, et al. Clinical implications of cardiac-mibg spect in the differentiation of parkinsonian syndromes[J]. J Clin Neurol, 2006, 2(1): 51-57.

[19] KASHIHARA K, OHNO M, KAWADA S, et al. Reduced cardiac uptake and enhanced washout of 123I-MIBG in pure autonomic failure occurs conjointly with Parkinson's disease and dementia with Lewy bodies[J]. J Nucl Med, 2006, 47(7): 1099-1101.

[20] RASCOVSKY K, HODGES J R, KIPPS C M, et al. Diagnostic criteria for the behavioral variant of frontotemporal dementia (bvFTD): current limitations and future directions [J]. Alzheimer Dis Assoc Disord, 2007, 21(4): S14-18.

[21] MCKEITH I G, DICKSON D W, LOWE J, et al. Diagnosis and management of dementia with Lewy bodies: third report of the DLB consortium [J]. Neurology, 2005, 65(12): 1863-1872.

[22] GILMAN S, WENNING G K, LOW P A, et al. Second consensus statement on the diagnosis of multiple system atrophy [J]. Neurology, 2008, 71(9): 670-676.

附录六 缩略词表

缩写	英文名称	中文名称
AD	Alzheimer's disease	阿尔茨海默病（老年痴呆症）
ALS	amyotrophic lateral sclerosis	肌萎缩侧索硬化
BR	midbrain raphe	中缝核
CBD	corticobasal degeneration	皮质基底节变性
CN	caudate nucleus	尾状核
DLB	dementia with Lewy bodies	路易体痴呆
ET	essential tremor	原发性震颤
FTLD	frontotemporal lobar degeneration	额颞叶变性
LN	lentiform nucleus	豆状核
MDD	major depression disorder	以抑郁为主要表现的疾病
Midbrain	midbrain area decrease (axial plan)	中脑
MSA	multiple system atrophy	多系统萎缩

续表

缩写	英文名称	中文名称
PD	Parkinson's disease	帕金森病
PDD	PD with dementia	帕金森病痴呆
PD-MCI	Parkinson's disease with mild cognitive impairment	帕金森病合并轻度认知功能障碍
PIGD	postural instability gait difficulty	姿势障碍型（帕金森病）
PSP-P	parkinsonism phenotype of progressive supranuclear palsy	以帕金森综合征为主要表型的进行性核上性麻痹
PSP-RS	classical Richardsonsyndrome of progressive supranuclear palsy	以经典理查森综合征为主要表型的进行性核上性麻痹
RLS	restless legs syndrome	不安腿综合征
RN	red nucleus	红核
SN	substantia nigra	黑质
TCS	transcranial sonography	经颅超声
TD	tremor dominate	震颤型（帕金森病）
TV	third ventricle	第三脑室
WD	Wilson disease	肝豆状核变性疾病

续表

缩写	英文名称	中文名称
	huntington disease	亨廷顿病
	indeterminate PD	中间型（帕金森病）
	Vascular parkinsonian syndromes	血管性帕金森综合征
	Primary Focal Dystonia	原发性肌张力障碍